COMMUNITY HEALTH

EDUCATION METHODS

A Practitioner's Guide

Edited By:

Robert J. Bensley, Ph.D.
Western Michigan University

Jodi Brookins-Fisher, Ph.D., C.H.E.S.
Central Michigan University

JONES AND BARTLETT PUBLISHERS
Sudbury, Massachusetts
BOSTON   TORONTO   LONDON   SINGAPORE

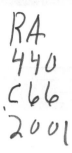

RA
440
C66
2001

World Headquarters
Jones and Bartlett Publishers
40 Tall Pine Drive
Sudbury, MA 01776
978-443-5000
info@jbpub.com
www.jbpub.com

Jones and Bartlett Publishers Canada
2406 Nikanna Road
Mississauga, ON L5C 2W6
CANADA

Jones and Bartlett Publishers International
Barb House, Barb Mews
London W6 7PA
UK

Library of Congress Catalog Card Number: 97-72291

ISBN: 0-7637-1601-4

Printed in the United States of America
03 02 01 00 99   10 9 8 7 6 5 4 3 2 1

Dedicated to an honored mentor, colleague, friend, and father . . .

This book is dedicated to **Loren B. Bensley, Jr.**, truly one of the purest health educators in the profession. Throughout his career, Dr. Bensley dedicated his life to health education; contributing ideals, morality, and a true sense of what the term "professionalism" means. He is one of the most respected professionals of our time and is commonly referred to by many as "the health educator's, health educator."

Much of this text is written and edited by those who, through having had the opportunity to study under the guidance of Dr. Bensley, continue to strive to uphold the level of professionalism that he empowered in them. In many ways, this book is a direct result of his teachings. It represents the ideals for which he stands, his commitment to the profession, and his un-wavering belief in the future generation of health education.

Contents

Chapter 1 **Community Health Assessment and Improvement**

Chapter 2 **Building Coalitions**

Chapter 3 **Conducting Focus Groups**

Preface

How many times have you heard the comment, "So what do you do as a health educator?" You respond with an answer such as, "Well, to be truthful, I work with populations and help them adopt certain behaviors and attitudes that are conducive to health." In response you hear, "Okay, sure. But what is it that you actually *do*?" No matter how hard you try to explain, the result is typically the same. Confusion. Bewilderment. Uncertainty. People want to understand but planning, programming, evaluating, and preventing disease are tough concepts to explain in real terms. What *do* we actually do as health educators?

The concepts and ideas presented in this book not only answers this question, they address *how* we do our jobs. It is a book about the methods we use as health educators—the ways in which we tell a story and empower others to seek healthy life-styles. It explains the basic tools that we need in order to communicate messages to those we are trying to serve, and provides us with an understanding of the skills we need to make a difference.

This text is unique in the sense that it is written *by* and *for* local health education practitioners. Rather than an "ivory towered" theoretical view, this book comes straight from the trenches, where *real* health education occurs. There are many academics who espouse well-versed ideas and solutions. They are eloquent in their approach and are brilliant in their thinking. This is not to say that these individuals are out-of-touch with reality. Quite the opposite is true. Most academicians we know are very knowledgeable about the issues they embrace, and have a thorough understanding of the factors that influence and impede effectiveness. They are developers, researchers, and theorists, and truly important to the advancement of the health education profession. This book, however, is not for them. It is for the health educator who is existing on a "shoestring" budget, attempting to implement strategies that the theorists and researchers have proven to work. It is for the overburdened practitioner who is working with multiple populations, across multiple settings, that are experiencing multiple problems. It is a guide to assist those on the front line of health education in completing their mission.

The contributing authors to this book have been or currently are living and breathing health education on a day-to-day basis. As such, they are experts in what they do. They provide a wisdom that cannot be found in the eloquent writings of academia. It is practical, useful, and adaptable knowledge garnered from years of experience in the State of Michigan. As you read through the text, you will find that almost every chapter contains insight, practical steps, techniques for success, and tips for overcoming barriers. It truly is a *practitioner's* guide. Use it. Follow it. *Make* a difference.

That is what a health educator does.

Robert J. Bensley, Ph.D.
Western Michigan University

Jodi Brookins-Fisher, Ph.D., C.H.E.S.
Central Michigan University

Acknowledgments

As with any project of this magnitude, there are numerous individuals whose contributions are usually "behind the scenes" but are paramount to its success. It is in part due to their efforts that this text has come to fruition.

First and foremost, we want to acknowledge the individual authors of this text for agreeing to contribute their experiences and knowledge related to community health education practices. Without them, this book would not exist. Their integrity, dedication, knowledge, patience, and understanding are definitely appreciated.

We also would like to acknowledge the efforts of many who had a part in creating, editing, and reviewing various parts of this text. In particular, we want to acknowledge the following: David Artley, Bill Bensley, Jim Bensley, Joan Bensley, Loren Bensley, Yasmina Bouraoui, Tody Casino, Jeff Cyzman, Laurie Fitzpatrick, Jackie Gilbert, George Lafkas, Jim Lewis, Dina Matt, Drew Reardon, Virginia Smith, Lori Stegmier, Tim Turton, Charles Wagner, and Balance Group Publishers.

The local Michigan community health educators who have shared offices with, served as mentors to, and collaborated on projects with the authors of this text deserve recognition for the role they have played in shaping the skills and experiences of the authors. The agencies for which the authors work and the populations that they serve also deserve credit for providing authors with opportunities to gain knowledge and practical experiences.

Finally, we acknowledge our families for their unwavering support during this project. Kathy, Kara, Katilee, Jack and Paul, we thank you for your patience, support, and understanding. Your unconditional belief and hope are what keep us going.

Author Biographies

Michelle Baukema, B.A.A., is currently employed as a Health Screener with the Washtenaw County Health Department, located in Ypsilanti, Michigan. Michelle previously served as a Tobacco Reduction Coalition Coordinator for a large metropolitan area, and gained extensive experience in community development, fund-raising, local and statewide legislative advocacy, and testifying at legislative hearings. Michelle has been a practicing health educator for the past seven years.

Leslie J. Bek, M.A., has served in many health education roles over the past 18 years, including Community Health Educator; Chief of the Division of Health Education, Planning and Evaluation; and Administrator of the Division of Community Health, Personal Health and Dental Health; all while at Marquette County Health Department, a rural health department located in the Upper Peninsula of Michigan. She has also served as an Adjunct Professor of Community Health at Northern Michigan University and is the owner of an independent health education consulting firm. Leslie has extensive experience working in community empowerment, having served in the capacity of convener, facilitator, leader, and member.

Robert J. Bensley, Ph.D., is currently employed by Western Michigan University where he serves as an Assistant Professor in the Health, Physical Education and Recreation Department and coordinates the Community Health Education program. Robert has spent most of his career focusing on building resilience and protective traits in at-risk youth, community development, and issues associated with professional preparation. Prior to his tenure in the health education profession, Robert was employed by IBM, where he served as a Systems Engineer providing technical assistance and technical systems planning to educational institutions, hospitals, and local government agencies.

Jodi Brookins-Fisher, Ph.D., C.H.E.S., has been a health educator for the past seven years and is currently an Assistant Professor in the Department of Health Promotion and Rehabilitation at Central Michigan University. An expert in diversity, Jodi has focused much of her research and service activities on multicultural issues. During her tenure as a health education professional, Jodi has developed a curriculum for teachers and school counselors regarding gay and lesbian youth issues, conducted sensitivity trainings for school district personnel, and taught diversity awareness courses at The University of Utah and Central Michigan University.

Lisa E. J. Clark, B.S., is a recent graduate of the Community Health Education program at Western Michigan University and is currently employed as the Member Services Director for the Safety Council for West Michigan. Prior to this position, she worked as a Migrant Outreach Worker for the Sparta Health Center, located in West Michigan.

Denise R. Cyzman, M.S., R.D., C.H.E.S., is the Chief of the Consultation and Certification Unit in the Diabetes, Dementia and Kidney Section, and the Assistant Director of the Michigan Diabetes Control Program, both of which are with the Michigan Department of Community Health. Denise's current duties involve management of unit staff and their responsibilities, including the Diabetes Outpatient Education Certification Program, the Diabetes Policy Advisory Committee, staff consultation to local agencies, contract management, and the Michigan Renal Disease Prevention and Education Program. Denise has worked in the health education field for the past 15 years. Her experience includes working in the capacity as both a staff and a supervisory health educator in city, county and state health departments, as well as in a hospital health promotion setting.

Susan B. Dusseau, M.A., C.H.E.S., is currently the Executive Director of the Midland Community Cancer Services, a United Way Agency located in Midland, Michigan. In addition to her administrative duties, she provides numerous community tobacco and cancer prevention services. Her grant writing experiences began with a proposal for state funds to provide county-wide substance abuse prevention services. Among her successful grant funded projects include extensive capital expansion, breast and cervical cancer screening outreach, patient assistance, expanded services to families of children with cancer, and tobacco reduction advocacy. Susan has been a practicing health educator for over 15 years.

Mary T. Gustas, Ed. Spec., has been Executive Director for the Safety Council for West Michigan for the past four years. Prior to this, she worked in higher education administration in Michigan and New Mexico, health care, the court system, and government as an aide for a Michigan State Representative. Mary has been working in various public relations and media positions for the past 19 years. She is also currently completing a Ph.D. in Applied Sociology at Western Michigan University.

John O. Nelson, M.P.A., C.H.E.S., is currently the Director of Program Planning and Evaluation at the Berrien County Health Department located in Benton Harbor, Michigan. He has previously served as a Health Educator, Substance Abuse Prevention Coordinator, Health Education Supervisor, and Health Promotion/Community Assessment Division Director for the

Berrien County Health Department, as well as an educator for the Planned Parenthood Association of Southwestern Michigan. As the Division Director of Health Promotion/Community Assessment, John had the opportunity to work with a staff, agency, and community that were dedicated to improving the health of Berrien County residents through needs assessment, prioritization, and enactment of a process that meets the standards of *Healthy People 2000*. John has been a practicing health educator for the past 16 years.

Jean M. Prout, *M.A.*, *C.H.E.S.*, is currently an adjunct instructor in the Department of Health Promotion and Rehabilitation and the Department of Human Environmental Studies at Central Michigan University. She is the founder of Lifelong Learning, Ltd., a health education consulting organization that provides educational workshops throughout Michigan. Jean is also an experienced grant writer, having received federal funding for five consecutive years. With more than 15 years experience in health education, Jean has chaired numerous committees, is well known for her work in program planning, and has received numerous awards for her dedication and commitment. She is currently working on a doctorate in Educational Leadership at Eastern Michigan University.

Beverly A. Riley, *M.A.*, is currently the Program Coordinator for Project ASSIST (American Stop Smoking Intervention Study), located in Kalamazoo, Michigan. For the past two years, a major focus of Beverly's position with Project ASSIST has been media advocacy. She currently supports the efforts of the Kalamazoo County Tobacco Reduction Coalition to reduce tobacco use through policy and media advocacy. Beverly has been a practicing health educator for the past seven years and has served as Project Manager for the Community Prevention Partnership in Kalamazoo, free-lance grant writer, community study consultant, and supervisor of programs for low-income families and individuals.

Lisa R. Rutherford, *M.A.*, *C.H.E.S.*, has been employed as a health educator and a health planner/evaluator for the past eight years. She has worked in rural and urban local public health departments, specializing in the areas of HIV/AIDS, coalition development and planning, and community assessment. Through this experience, Lisa has planned and coordinated a variety of focus group projects, as well as conducted analysis and reporting of focus group data. Currently, she is a consultant for development, planning, and evaluation of health initiatives for various agencies, including local public health. She is also currently a Community Technical Assistant to community-based coalitions funded through the Michigan Abstinence Partnership.

Shelly E. Schadewald, M.A., C.H.E.S., has worked in various areas within the health education profession over the last 10 years, including worksite health promotion, program marketing and management, and has spent the last seven years in pregnancy prevention. Shelly is currently the Coordinator of the Michigan Abstinence Partnership of the Michigan Department of Community Health, an award winning initiative that currently leads the nation in making abstinence a public health issue. Shelly also has served as President of the Great Lakes Chapter of the Society for Public Health Education.

Stephanie Sikora, B.S., C.H.E.S., is a health educator currently employed by the Kent County Health Department located in Grand Rapids Michigan where she works with violence prevention issues. Previously, she served as the materials coordinator for the health education section of the health department and was responsible for the quality and accuracy of printed health education materials.

Heather M. Stys, B.S., is currently pursuing a Master's degree in Health Education and Health Promotion at Central Michigan University. In the past four years, she has worked as a community health educator at a tri-county health department and as a health promotion coordinator in a university setting. Heather is an expert speaker and has presented various health topics to over 3,000 people.

Richard M. Tooker, M.D., M.P.H., is a practicing Family Physician, with training in Public Health and Epidemiology, and currently serves as the Chief Medical Officer and Examiner for the Kalamazoo County Human Services Department, in Kalamazoo, Michigan. He is also the Medical Director for the Branch-Hillsdale-St. Joseph District Health Department and the Chief Medical Examiner for the Van Buren County Public Health Department, both located in Michigan. Richard has spent most of his career in public health, beginning as a environmental field epidemiologist. Although a physician by training, Richard has been intimately involved in public health education endeavors, serving as Chairman of the Kalamazoo County Tobacco Reduction Coalition and the Kalamazoo County Health Promotion Committee.

Mikelle D. Whitt, M.A., has worked as a Public Health Consultant for the Tobacco Section of the Michigan Department of Community Health for the past eight years, where she has engaged in providing technical assistance and support to local tobacco reduction coalitions, contract management for a project funded by the National Cancer Institute, coordinating statewide tobacco reduction trainings, and acting as a resource on tobacco related laws and policy development. Prior experience includes six years as a health educator in two local health departments promoting child safety programs, building local adolescent pregnancy prevention coalitions, fund raising, and grant writing.

Foreword

In a recent article by Cheryl Jackson on issues related to behavioral science theory and principles for practice in health education, she noted:[1]

> *Experience engenders knowledge of the people, knowledge of the problem, and knowledge of the social system in which the problem occurs. Experience engenders trust, familiarity, cultural sensitivity and political awareness—all essential to successful intervention. Optimally, practitioners can draw upon their theoretical and experiential knowledge as they plan, implement and evaluate health education programs.*

Community Health Education Methods: A Practitioner's Guide is a unique example of drawing on the wealth of experience from the health education practitioners in the State of Michigan to indeed inform the field in many of the basic essential skills associated with community health education.

Having spent most of my life and at least half of my career in Michigan, it is a great pleasure to join my two friends and colleagues in providing opening remarks for this text. As one who has spent a great deal of time around the country working at many levels in health education, I have always been proud of the strong and powerful health education heritage and expertise that abounds in Michigan. There is a strong history of health education leadership, research, professional preparation, and, most importantly, practice. The editors and authors of this text represent many of those key elements.

This text includes what many of us call the "nuts and bolts," or basic elements, of a local health educator's tool box. The strength of this book is that the chapters are written by local practitioners—those who are on the front line and enmeshed in health education activities on a day-to-day basis. The authors have combined their extensive practical experience with their knowledge of the professional literature to provide practical advise and guidance for fellow practitioners.

It is imperative that health education practitioners at all levels of preparation and practice settings strive for excellence and quality in what they do. This text provides practitioners with the necessary skills that allow this to happen.

Brick Lancaster, M.A., C.H.E.S.
Associate Director for Health Education
Practice and Policy
Division of Adult and Community Health
Centers for Disease Control and Prevention
Atlanta, GA

Reference

1.   Jackson, C. (1997). Behavioral science theory and principles for practice in health education. *Health Education Research, Theory & Practice, 12*(1), 143-150.

Chapter 1

COMMUNITY HEALTH ASSESSMENT AND IMPROVEMENT

John O. Nelson, M.P.A., C.H.E.S.

Author's Comments: *The activities associated with community health assessment and improvement exemplify many of the tasks and responsibilities of a health educator. This chapter describes major components of the process and is written with the goal that the reader, when given the opportunity to participate in the process, will have sufficient insight needed to succeed.*

Community health and assessment is a challenge! Being involved in community health assessment and improvement over the past six years, I have been amazed by the energy that revolves around the identification and prioritization of community health problems and the development and implementation of strategies to address these problems. Through the collaboration and partnerships that are created as a result of this process, communities are able to see real change in relation to the problems at hand.

Naturally, the entire process requires planning, commitment, patience, resources, communication, and trust. The health educator that recognizes this (and has the tools to proceed) will be prepared to actively participate in and/or facilitate community health assessment and improvement.

INTRODUCTION

In 1988, the Institute of Medicine (IOM) of the National Academy of Sciences published *The Future of Public Health*, a landmark report that provided direction for a shift in the core functions of public health agencies from clinical services, to assessment, policy development, and assurance.[1] In order to adequately address the function of community health assessment, the IOM recommended that every public health agency regularly and systematically collect, analyze, and make available information on the health of the community, including statistics on health status, community health needs, and epidemiological studies of health problems. These functions are necessary to undertake the mission of public health: To assure conditions in society in which people can be healthy.

This chapter focuses on the process of community health assessment and improvement, including identification of goals, participants involved, models, and practical steps. Also included are tips and techniques for success, barriers to community health assessment and improvement, strategies for overcoming barriers, and expected outcomes.

Community health assessment and improvement can be defined as a dynamic process undertaken to identify the health needs of the community, enabling the establishment of health priorities and collaborative action planning, that is directed at improving community health. The assessment draws upon both quantitative and qualitative data specified to the entire target population.[2] It specifically involves the previously mentioned core functions of public health: Assessment, policy development, and assurance. During the community health assessment and improvement process, the local health department carries out the *assessment* function by assisting the community in analyzing its health, and investigating the occurrence of the health effects and health hazards in the community.[3] The function of *policy development* is addressed as the local health department assists the community in setting priorities among health needs, identifying resources in the community, and developing plans and policies to address priority health needs.[3] The *assurance* function of public health occurs within the community health assessment and improvement process as the local health department participates with the community in developing organizational structures and managing community resources to address priority health needs. This includes informing and educating the public, implementing programs and assuring the delivery of services based on identified needs, evaluating programs, and providing quality assurance.

In many communities, the definition of community health assessment and improvement has been expanded beyond merely the gathering of health data. This definition has been broadened to include a community partnership between public and private health care systems and community health members for improving the health of the community. It is these partnerships that meld the core functions of public health. The local health department is centrally involved with each function in the community health assessment and improvement process as part of these partnerships.

COMMUNITY HEALTH ASSESSMENT AND IMPROVEMENT GOALS

The documents *Healthy People: The Surgeon General's Report on Health Promotion and Disease Prevention* (later revised to *Promoting Health/Preventing Disease: Objectives for the Nation*) established a national agenda to prevent unnecessary disease and disability and to achieve a better quality of life for all Americans.[4,5] The current agenda, as described in *Healthy People 2000: National Health Promotion and Disease Prevention Objectives*, offers a vision for the new century, characterized by significant reductions in preventable death and disability, enhanced quality of life, and greatly reduced disparities in the health status of populations.[6]

A collaborative effort between the U.S. Department of Health and Human Services, 22 expert working groups, the IOM, and a national consortium of nearly 300 national membership organizations and all state health departments, developed the *Healthy People 2000* objectives to measure progress in addressing U.S. health issues.[7] The purpose of *Healthy People 2000* is to commit the nation to the attainment of three broad goals that include (1) increasing the span of healthy life for all U.S. citizens, (2) reducing health disparities among U.S. citizens, and (3) achieving access for preventive services for all U.S. citizens. The report includes objectives to achieve by the year 2000 organized into 22 priority areas. The first 21 areas are organized into the three broad categories of health promotion, health protection, and preventive services. The remaining priority area encompasses surveillance and data systems (see Table 1-1). *Healthy People 2000* provides benchmarks (objectives) for local communities and states to choose from when selecting priority health problems to address for community health improvement. The objectives are not federal standards or requirements, but simply guides for communities.

Healthy People 2000 also includes 326 objectives to improve the health of U.S. citizens by the beginning of the 21st century. The achievement of these objectives is dependent in part on the ability of health agencies at all levels of government to assess objective progress. To permit comparison, procedures have been developed and disseminated among federal, state, and local agencies for collecting comparable data.[8]

Objectives are designed to measurably improve the public health status of millions of Americansæone city, town, or county at a timeæby the end of the 20th century. The challenge is to meet these objectives with limited financial resources and personnel by marshaling community resources and support.[9]

The State of Michigan, as an example, has modeled its objectives after *Healthy People 2000* in the document *Healthy Michigan 2000*. First published in 1993, *Healthy Michigan 2000* established priority areas and goals and objectives related to each priority. It is a strategic plan that guides statewide actions to address the most pressing health needs of Michigan residents.[10] In summary, the goals of community health assessment and improvement are to systematically implement a process to improve the health status of the citizens of a particular geographic area. This process begins with the collection of health data, choosing quantifiable health benchmarks, and the identification of health priorities that need to be addressed.

Table 1-1. *Healthy People 2000* Priority Areas

Health Promotion

1.   Physical Activity and Fitness
2.   Nutrition
3.   Tobacco
4.   Alcohol and Other Drugs
5.   Family Planning
6.   Mental Health and Mental Disorders
7.   Violent and Abusive Behavior
8.   Educational and Community-Based Programs

Health Protection

9.   Unintentional Injuries
10. Occupational Safety and Health
11. Environmental Health
12. Food and Drug Safety
13. Oral Health

Preventive Services

14. Maternal and Infant Health
15. Heart Disease and Stroke
16. Cancer
17. Diabetes and Chronic Disabling Conditions
18. HIV Infection
19. Sexually Transmitted Diseases
20. Immunization and Infectious Diseases
21. Clinical Preventive Services

Surveillance and Data Systems

22. Surveillance and Data Systems

COMMUNITY PARTICIPANTS

Successful community health assessment and improvement efforts depend upon solid partnerships between public and private sectors, governmental and nongovernmental agencies, business and labor, consumers, and providers.[10] Partners in the community assessment and improvement process should include the local health department, hospitals, community-based health care organizations, the area agency on aging, social services, local foundations, representatives from education, and neighborhood improvement associations.

Community coalitions (e.g., those established for teenage pregnancy prevention, tobacco reduction, violence prevention, substance abuse prevention, and cardiovascular disease risk reduction), are ideal partners for community health assessment and improvement as they are collaborative groups of community individuals and agencies that work together toward a common purpose. Including existing coalitions in the health assessment process will provide valuable input and involvement in improving the health of the population.

COMMUNITY HEALTH ASSESSMENT AND IMPROVEMENT MODELS

Several models have been developed to assist in the community health assessment and improvement process, more notably the Assessment Protocol for Excellence in Public Health (APEX*PH*)[11] and the Planned Approach to Community Health (PATCH).[12] Hybrid models, based upon standard models, have also been utilized.

APEX*PH* was developed by the Centers for Disease Control and Prevention as a tool for local health departments to use in data collection and community organization efforts. APEX*PH* improves the system of public health in a community by enhancing the community's capacity to perform the core functions of assessment, policy development, and assurance. The APEX*PH* model also encourages and strengthens the ability of the local public health agency to provide leadership in the development and implementation of a community health plan.[9]

APEX*PH* is a three-part process: (1) Organizational Capacity Assessment, (2) The Community Process, and (3) Completing the Cycle. *Organizational Capacity Assessment* consists of an internal review of a local health department. This component aids in assessing a health department's basic administrative capacity and its capacity to undertake the second step (The Community Process), and is conducted by the health department director and a team of key staff members. *The Community Process,* is intended to be a more public endeavor, involving key members of the community, as well as department staff, in assessing the health of the community and identifying the role of the health department in relation to community strengths and health problems. During this phase, both objective health data and the community's perceptions of community health problems are utilized. *Completing the Cycle,* integrates the plans developed during the first two phases of the process into the ongoing activities of a health department and the community served. Focus is directed toward policy development, assurance, monitoring, and evaluation of plans developed in the first two phases.[11]

PATCH is a process that enables communities to plan, implement, and evaluate programs designed for reducing the burden of disease. PATCH is a community health promotion method that will increase a community's capacity to organize and mobilize members, collect and use local data, set health priorities, select and implement appropriate interventions, and perform process and impact evaluation.[9] Although it can be employed as a generic planning/implementation process, it is primarily geared toward chronic disease prevention and health promotion programs. This model is often employed to affect and change public policy and environmental factors, as well as individual decisions regarding life-styles and behavior in the community.[9]

Several other national models and reports have been prepared and published over the past 20 years that provide a starting point for addressing community health assessment and improvement. In particular: *Model Standards for Community Health Services*,[4] and *Healthy Communities 2000: Model Standards*.[13] These models and reports identify a wide range of problems for which strategies and interventions exist to significantly improve a community's health status. They also recognize the need for public and private collaboration; emphasize the importance of community participation, local leadership, and strong intergovernmental relations; and assert the need to plan and evaluate public health efforts on the basis of objective statistical data.[11]

The *Healthy Communities 2000* model encourages local public health agencies to involve local leaders and decision makers in determining their own public health priorities and to establish objectives that are compatible with the national objectives and targets.[7] This model is based on an 11-step approach (see Table 1-2).

STEPS TO IMPLEMENTING A COMMUNITY HEALTH ASSESSMENT AND IMPROVEMENT PROCESS

Individual states have modified and used the above models for implementation in local communities. For example, the State of Michigan has instituted an eight-step model for community health assessment and improvement that is based on the *Healthy Communities 2000* standards. The steps associated with this process include (1) defining the community, (2) organizing the community to participate in community health assessment and improvement, (3) assessing health needs and determining available community health resources, (4) determining community priorities, (5) selecting objectives, (6) developing intervention strategies, (7) developing and implementing a plan of action, and (8) monitoring and evaluating efforts. For the purposes of this chapter, this model will be used to illustrate the community health assessment and improvement process.

Defining the Community

Each local health department should develop partnerships with key community agencies, community leaders, interest groups, and community members. Identifying key people and organizations to involve in a partnership effort is fundamental to a local health department's success and an essential part of community leadership. Although key individuals and agencies differ for each community, many communities include representatives from hospitals and other health care agencies, community-based organizations, educational institutions, social services, foundations, neighborhood associations, and local government. Typical leaders include members of City Council and school boards, Superintendent of Schools, influential church leaders, Chief of police, and presidents of local service clubs. The local health department should conduct an assessment of the community's organizational and power structures either on a formal or informal basis as part of its strategy in developing partnerships.[9] Including the community's organizational and power structures in the community assessment and improvement process will help ensure success.

Organizing Community Participation

Health is not a commodity that is given. It must be generated from within. Similarly, health action cannot be an effort imposed from outside and foreign to the people; rather it must be a response of the community to the problems that the people in the community perceive, carried out in a way that is acceptable to them and properly supported by an adequate infrastructure. - Halfdan Mahler.

The local health agency should convene community groups for assessing health needs, addressing health problems, and assisting in the coordination of responsibilities. Community leaders are needed to create and strengthen relationships between private and public sector groups. Broader communication efforts will facilitate coordinated actions that could not be realized through single agency efforts. A constituency of individuals concerned about community health that can advocate for resources and for the attention of elected officials, is increasingly essential to local health agency success.[9]

At the community level, local public health departments should facilitate the process that engages all stakeholders with an interest in community health. Stakeholders include consumers, providers, businesses, public and private agencies, and other individuals and organizations vested in the future of the community. Broad participation should be sought to assure representation of all segments of the community in building health from a grass roots effort.[10]

During this step of the community health assessment and improvement process, important questions need to be considered: Are the partners in the process reflective of changes taking place in the private and public health care system? Is the community health assessment and improvement

Table 1-2. The *Healthy Communities 2000* Model

1.   Assessing and determining the role of one's agency.
2.   Assessing the lead health agency's organizational capacity.
3.   Developing an agency plan to build the necessary organizational capacity.
4.   Assessing the community's organizational and power structures.
5.   Organizing the community to build a stronger constituency for public health and establish a partnership for public health.
6.   Assessing health needs and available community resources.
7.   Determining local priorities.
8.   Selecting outcome and process objectives that are compatible with local priorities and the *Healthy People 2000* objectives.
9.   Developing community-wide intervention strategies.
10. Developing and implementing a plan of action.
11. Monitoring and evaluating the effort on a continuing basis.

process integrated with other community planning processes or the human services coordinating body?

Each community will be unique in the roles played by the various partners. For example, the local health department may be a leader, convener, facilitator, or participant. Hospitals may actively lead or participate in the process. Community foundations may serve as conveners, participants, or major funding agencies for the interventions developed.[10]

Some community health assessment and improvement initiatives have engaged the community by establishing an organizational structure comprised of a steering committee and several task forces. The function of the steering committee is to provide direction for the entire community process and assure needed resources are available for carrying out the community assessment plan. Task forces, comprised of agency and community representatives, are responsible for developing and implementing the action steps for community health improvement. A task force is usually facilitated by a local health educator. Therefore, it is imperative that health educators involved in the community assessment and improvement project have strong group facilitation skills. Upon completion of the task force interventions, a report should be submitted to the steering committee.

Assessing Needs and Determining Resources

A community health assessment will provide the information needed to identify a community's most critical health problems. The community health assessment and improvement process should include both formal and informal data collection. It should identify the perceptions and values of community leaders, groups, agencies, individuals, and health department staff about health priorities for the community. The effort should also examine pertinent health data and survey information to identify and verify the extent of major health problems and the level of risk for subpopulations. An inventory of available community resources should be developed.[9]

The assessment of health needs can be conducted through a variety of means. Health data is readily available at the federal, state, and local levels. At the federal level, the National Center for Health Statistics of the Centers for Disease Control and Prevention is the nation's principal health statistics agency. Its mission is to provide statistical information to guide actions and policies to improve the health of Americans. At the state level, community health profiles by county and region may be available. In Michigan, the *Community Health Profiles Project* provides each community in the state with a basic description of its health.[14] Other states may have similar information.

Other sources of information may also be obtained. These include behavioral risk factor surveys, critical health indicators, community maps, and community scans.

Behavioral risk factor surveys are a primary source of a community's behavioral risk. Data from these surveys are invaluable in helping to assist in predicting the future health of the community. Many states participate in the Behavior Risk Factor Survey (BRFS) which provides statewide population-based estimates of the prevalence of behavior risk factors among adults. The BRFS is a statewide telephone survey of a representative sample of residents 18 years of age and older. For instance, in Michigan, the survey consisted of approximately 200 interviews each month for an annual total of nearly 2,400 interviews.[10] Health issues in a BRFS will include such topics as access to health care, perceived health status, cigarette smoking status, weight status, diet and physical activity, and cancer screening.

Critical health indicators are a select group of health factors that gauge the health of a geographical area over time (e.g., infant mortality rates, teenage pregnancy rates, and cancer rates). The indicators are often used to compare one geographic area to another in terms of key aspects of life expectancy, health risk behaviors, disease and disability, causes of death, health care, and social factors.

Community mapping identifies community assets and accessibility. Community assets include health care agencies, community-based organizations, educational institutions, public transportation, and other resources that exist in the community. Assets mapping is an innovative approach for describing the health of the community from a positive perspective. Indi-

> *If we could first know where we are and whither we are tending, we could then better judge what to do and how to do it.* - Abraham Lincoln

vidual assets (e.g., skills, interests, and experience), association assets (e.g., interest groups), and institution assets (e.g., facilities, employment, and education) should be identified. Access to health resources needs to be considered as well, comparing the location, affordability, and limitations of resources to the community. Communities often feel that they have been "over needs-assessed" by agencies, foundations, and academic institutions. Rather than focusing on the community's problems, assets-based mapping allows a community to highlight resources and successful initiatives as a catalyst for additional community improvement.

Community scanning is the process of reviewing literature pertinent to the community being assessed. The community scan will provide information on what has already been learned through previous assessments, and will point out the critical issues that the particular community faces. Examples of community scans include the U.S. Census; annual reports prepared by cities, counties, and states; public health data; and vital statistics.

Determining Community Priorities

Local communities commonly face an increasing range of pressing health problems that must be met with limited, or decreasing, resources. To allocate these resources, communities must establish priorities among the multitude of problems. For this difficult task, communities will need a process that is fair, reasonable, and easy to use. The process should ensure that all health problems will be addressed in a similar manner.

As with all steps in community health assessment and improvement, establishing local priorities, such as addressing heart disease, cancer, stroke, infant mortality, teenage pregnancy, immunization status of children, or a wide variety of other health issues, should involve major health agencies, organizations, and key interest groups and individuals. Information gathered from a community health assessment is intended to aid in determining local priorities. Selection of priorities should be decided by negotiation among community groups, resulting in a set of priority health problems to be targeted for community action.[9]

The most commonly used methods for determining priorities involves identifying the size and seriousness of each community health problem and the effectiveness of available interventions. For example, the Pickett and Hanlon method is a way of setting priorities and includes the following main components: (1) Rating the size of the health problem, (2) rating the seriousness of the health problem, (3) rating the health problems for the effectiveness of available interventions, and (4) applying the *Propriety, Economics, Acceptability, Resources,* and *Legality* (PEARL) test. Priority scores are calculated from the numbers recorded for size, seriousness, and effectiveness of intervention for each health problem. Once priority scores have been recorded for all health problems, a priority rank will be assigned to each.[15]

Additional opportunities for encouraging community involvement and achieving input include focus groups, community forums, and interviews and surveys. Focus groups provide an excellent means of encouraging community involvement. They are a powerful mechanism for learning the perceptions, experiences, values, and beliefs of community members regarding health status and health care. Participation in focus groups can be increased by offering several different sessions at various times and dates, and through using a moderator who is sensitive to both cultural and linguistic differences (see Chapter 3, "Conducting Focus Groups").

Community forums seek information directly from community members. Forums offer an opportunity for community members to raise concerns and become involved in developing strategies. Forums should also be held at convenient times and locations.

Interviews and surveys help to understand the perspectives, experiences, aspirations, values, and strengths of community members. All surveys and interviews should be conducted in a setting in which the individual feels comfortable.

Selecting Objectives

Healthy Communities 2000 can be used to negotiate and select appropriate goals and measurable outcome objectives for resolving community health problems. During this step of the community health assessment and improvement process, several important questions may be considered such as:

- Who decides what the objectives will be?

- Have both process and outcome objectives been identified that reflect the priorities of the local community?

- Are the objectives measurable and within a time frame?

- Are the objectives comparable to national or state objectives or a state planning document?

Establishing measurable, time-framed process and outcome objectives will provide the structure for a community to develop an action plan and monitor progress. Improvement can be made only when the community knows what it wants to achieve and how the community intends to achieve it. Local progress can also be measured by comparison of local community objectives to *Healthy People 2000* and the state's baseline objectives and targets.

Developing Intervention Strategies

Developing community-wide interventions will provide the means to achieve selected community goals and objectives. Once interventions have been selected, responsibilities should be assigned so that the activities can be distributed and coordinated among the participating community's agencies and organizations.[9] It may be beneficial to consider the following questions at this phase:

- Can implementation of the strategies developed by the community health improvement partners be expected to contribute to achievement of the objective?

- Do the strategies have a community-wide focus rather than an agency or organization focus?

- Have the strategies been incorporated into the work plans of related community initiatives or organizations?

Strategies that have a community-wide focus will be more likely to involve multiple agencies, organizations, and individuals in the implementation of the strategy. An example community-wide focus strategy would be an immunization registry that provides access to information regarding the immunization status of children in a particular geographic area. The registry would be linked to critical local and regional agencies, such as health departments, private physicians' offices, and hospitals.

Strategies that are narrowly focused may be appropriate as action steps for individual agencies or organizations. An example of a narrowly focused intervention is the development and distribution of a low-fat cookbook intended to reduce cardiovascular disease.

Developing and Implementing a Plan of Action

Success will depend on developing and executing a plan of action to implement intervention activities and services. Establishing time lines, and assigning responsibilities for activities and services, are essential parts of this process.[9] Likelihood for success may be enhanced in the implementation phase by (1) identifying each of the necessary action steps, (2) assigning

> *Whatever you can do, or dream you can, begin it. Boldness has genius, power, and magic in it.* - Johann Wolfgang van Goethe

responsibility for plan of action or action steps, (3) committing needed resources, and (4) distributing plans of action across community partners.

Using the media allows for community awareness, and increases the potential for commitment and involvement in the community health assessment and improvement process. By forming a proactive versus reactive position, the assessment team will be able to take full advantage of any opportunities for media exposure. For example, the project can institute regular press releases about activities. This will keep the press informed on a regular basis, and convey information about specific issues the team may want publicized.

Monitoring and Evaluating Efforts

In the long term, the achievement of improved health status will attest to the effectiveness of community efforts. In the short term, achievement of local process objectives will show movement toward improved health status, if effective interventions have been selected. For example, new services, enhancement of existing services, improved community linkages for coordinating efforts, and enhanced staff skills and morale, provide evidence of success.[9] During this step, several questions need to be considered:

- Is evaluation an ongoing, integral part of the process?

- Have performance measures been established for the community's process and outcome objectives and the community health assessment process in general?

- Are evaluation results broadly communicated?

- Are evaluation results being used to refine the community's objectives, strategies, and action plan?

STRATEGIES FOR OVERCOMING BARRIERS

Many potential barriers inhibit the process of a community health assessment and improvement project. Primary barriers surround the issues of governance and the leveraging of resources. Governance is the power to control decisions and resources. Leveraging issues include those associated with (1) recognizing and using community assets, (2) collaboration, and (3) sustaining involvement and commitment[16] (See Tables 1-3 and 1-4).

Strategies for overcoming the barriers to successful implementation of a community health assessment and improvement project include (1) identifying key people and keeping them involved, (2) building consensus, (3) keeping the community informed through networking and marketing, (4) maximizing resources, and (5) consultation. Reassessment of these strategies should occur at each phase of the community health assessment and improvement process to provide an opportunity for participants to avoid or minimize barriers.

Identifying key people in the community assessment and improvement process is important. Potential sources for key representatives may include elected officials or members of various agency governing boards or community-based funding sources. The expanded representatives may offer a different perspective from program administrators and may have a positive influence on decisions.

Building consensus may be achieved through the identification and clarification of the purpose of community health assessment and improvement, and effective communication of this purpose with participants. Community assessment and improvement participants need a succinct vision and mutual understanding of health and larger social issues. Building consensus also requires defining the authority of the governing body, how decisions will be made, and whether decisions will determine funding allocations.

Networking keeps the community informed by providing opportunities for the community health assessment and improvement participants

Table 1-3. Barriers Associated with Governance

Involvement and Commitment

1. Reluctance of community political and financial power brokers to "really" participate in the process.
2. Community apathy, demonstrated by a lack of participation or interest.
3. The challenge of fostering and supporting diverse participation in community governance.
4. A lack of effective leadership for positive changes.

Communication

5. A lack of clarity of purpose.
6. Differences in organizational and individual cultures.
7. A lack of awareness of personal vested interest.
8. A lack of acceptance or support of community values.
9. Difficulties in coordination of diverse stakeholders.

Structure

10. Unresolved questions that surround authority, legal status, and control.
11. Resistance to sharing resources.
12. Risks and responsibilities across traditional organizational boundaries.
13. Unresolved questions which revolve around the redefining of public and private partnerships.

to exchange ideas and share strategies and insights regarding challenges associated with community-based health issues. The local community and other communities alike will benefit from networking connections.

Marketing of a community health assessment and improvement project provides increased awareness and appreciation for community health issues. Increased community awareness may contribute to additional involvement during the development and implementation of the community plan. Marketing strategies include articulating to stakeholders (e.g., hospitals, businesses, the general public) how a healthier community benefits all people. Use of the "broken record" technique (constantly emphasizing the benefits and strengths of collaboration) may result in increased participation. Marketing can also be used to show progress by using the media to provide feedback to the community regarding community improvement successes.

Maximizing resources can be accomplished by initially developing a resource inventory. Resources should be broadly defined to include the money, ideas, time, and energy of various groups. Maximization of resources

Table 1-4. Barriers Associated with Leveraging

Community Assets
1. No agency or body taking the lead to secure additional resources.
2. Difficulty in justifying who should receive the resources when these are available.
3. A lack of sharing assets by stakeholders due to fear of risk and failure.
4. The perception of change from simply sharing information, to sharing resources among individuals and agencies.

Collaboration
5. Benefits and incentives have not been articulated, or are not clearly seen.
6. Territorial attitudes and competition have bred distrust.
7. Change is perceived as threatening, especially in an environment of diminishing resources.
8. Participants have agendas that may not be in the best interest of the community.
9. An inability to keep participants focused on unity and the common good exists.

Sustaining Involvement and Commitment
10. All segments of the community are not involved.
11. Community members are not convinced of problems and the need to address these problems.
12. The process is time consuming and gratification to participants is delayed.
13. Progress is difficult to demonstrate.

can be achieved through ensuring that each organization will make a commitment to their contributions.

Consultation with a nonparticipant in the local assessment process allows for additional technical assistance. Futurists and other consultants can provide a perspective for the local assessment process of similar collaborative efforts in other communities. In addition, a consultant may be able to identify the root cause of barriers, as well as provide recommendations on ameliorating barriers.[16]

EXPECTED OUTCOMES

The expected outcomes of community health assessment and improvement include improved health in a community, increased partnering of health care service organizations, and a shared sense of improved general well-being. *Healthy People 2000* objectives can serve as a guide or standard to measure the expected outcomes of community health assessment and improvement. These objectives provide outcome objectives to compare the health of the local community to that of the state or nation. Outcome measures may be related to morbidity and mortality, changes in health behaviors, and other similar indicators.

In addition, expected outcomes may be measured in terms of process objectives. These objectives may include increased collaboration or new partnerships formed in communities, anecdotal examples of positive health behaviors, and other related examples of improved health.

CONCLUSION

Community health assessment and improvement is a process that includes assessing the health needs and resources of the community, investigating the occurrence of health effects and hazards of the community, and analyzing the determinants of identified health needs. In this chapter, the definition of community health assessment and improvement was expanded to include the functions of policy development and assurance. Therefore, community health assessment and improvement is a process that engages the community in the identification of priority health problems or issues and in the development and implementation of interventions that are intended to address these problems or issues. The process is implemented for the purpose of improving the health of the community, region, state or nation.

References

1. Institute of Medicine. (1988). *The future of public health*. Washington, DC: National Academy Press.

2. Michigan Public Health Institute. (1995). *Community health profile training guidebook, 1995*. Okemos, MI: Author.

3. Michigan Health Officers Association, & Michigan Association of Local Public Health. (1993). *Promoting healthy Michigan communities: The role of public health in health reform*. Lansing, MI: Author.

4. Department of Health and Human Services. (1979). *Healthy people: Surgeon General's report on health promotion and disease prevention*. Washington, DC: U.S. Government Printing Office.

5. Department of Health and Human Services. (1980). *Promoting health/preventing disease: Objectives for the nation*. Washington, DC: U.S. Government Printing Office.

6. Department of Health and Human Services. (1991). *Healthy People 2000: National health promotion and disease prevention objectives* (DHHS Publication No. PHS 91-50212). Washington, DC: U.S. Government Printing Office.

7. Michigan Primary Care Association. (1996*). Primary health care: Profile of Michigan data book, June, 1996*. East Lansing, MI: Author.

8. Department of Health and Human Services. (1997). *Healthy People 2000 statistical notes, operational definitions for year 2000 objectives: Priority area 20, immunization and infectious diseases* (DHHS Publication No. PHS 97-1237). Hyattsville, MD: U.S. Government Printing Office.

9. American Public Health Association. (1993*). The guide to implementing model standards: Eleven steps toward a healthy community*. Washington, DC: Author.

10. Michigan Department of Community Health. (1996). *Healthy Michigan 2000: Preliminary strategic plan*. (2nd ed.). Lansing, MI: Author.

11. National Association of County Health Officials. (1991). *APEXPH: Assessment protocol for excellence in public health*. Washington, DC: Author.

12. Department of Health and Human Services. (1992). *The planned approach to community health: A guide for the local coordinator*. Atlanta, GA: Author.

13. American Public Health Association. (1991). *Healthy communities 2000: Model standards— Guidelines for community attainment of the year 2000 national objectives*. (3rd ed.). Washington, DC: National Academy Press.

14. Michigan Public Health Institute. (1996). *Community health profiles project: Framework for studying health care services in Michigan*. Okemos, MI: Author.

15. Pickett, G. E., & Hanlon, J. J. (1990). *Public Health Administration and Practice* (9th ed.). St. Louis: Mosby.

16. Michigan Department of Community Health. (1996). *Michigan community health assessment forum V: Proceedings—Sustaining an ongoing community health assessment*. Lansing, MI: Author.

Chapter 2

BUILDING COALITIONS

Mikelle D. Whitt, M.A.

Author's Comments: *Having been involved with coalitions at both the local and state level over the past 12 years, I have found coalition development and maintenance to be very challenging and rewarding. Working with coalitions has been insightful in relation to community organizing, local and state politics, interagency collaboration, and media relations. The most rewarding part, personally, has been in expanding networks to include the people and agencies who I have collaborated with on coalitions over the years. Also rewarding is knowing that coalition efforts reach so many more people and reap much greater benefit than an individual health educator could hope to achieve.*

This chapter has been written using a compilation of many past personal experiences, ideas gleaned from others, and the wisdom and advice of national experts. I hope that this information will help guide you in your efforts to develop and maintain a productive community coalition.

Always remember, the key to success is to think big about which groups and individuals to invite to join your coalition effort, and about what the coalition might possibly accomplish. Most importantly though, keep a good sense of humor and celebrate your "wins" along the way!

INTRODUCTION

A coalition is a temporary alliance of individuals and agencies working towards a common goal. It is different from other types of committees in that a structured arrangement for collaboration between organizations exists in which all members work together toward a common purpose. As an action-oriented group, a coalition focuses on reducing or preventing a community problem by (1) analyzing the problem, (2) identifying and implementing solutions, and (3) creating social change. More specifically, coalition functions include planning, advocacy, delivery of services, promoting public awareness, promoting risk reduction, conducting professional education, networking, building partnerships, and creating community change.[1]

Coalitions promote community change by serving as an effective and efficient forum for the exchange of knowledge, ideas, and strategies.

Through coalitions, individuals and organizations may become involved in new, broader issues without carrying the sole responsibility for dealing with the issues. Additional benefits of a coalition include the following:[2]

- Demonstrating and developing community support or concern for issues.
- Maximizing the power of individuals and groups through collective action.
- Preventing "reinventing the wheel."
- Improving trust and communication among community agencies.
- Mobilizing talents, resources, and strategies.
- Building strength and cohesiveness by connecting individual activists.
- Building a constituency.

Local health organizations can form or join coalitions to augment their limited resources of staff, time, talent, equipment, supplies, materials, contacts, and influence. Joining with other agencies and individuals can be beneficial to an organization, giving it expanded access to printing services, media coverage, marketing services, meeting space, community residents, influential people, postage, personnel, community and professional networks, and expertise.[1]

A coalition can be a very efficient means of instituting social change. Central to the coalition's effectiveness in bringing about change is the ability to work on a problem from a number of fronts by many people. There is no single approach for community change that is as effective as a broad-based coalition effort that provides the means for multiple strategies and involves key community individuals.[2]

COMMUNITY ORGANIZING

Traditional health education and prevention is only one small piece of a comprehensive community campaign. Health education has typically focused on health educators as teachers and agents of change for personal health habits. The process often involves organizing educational events, teaching classes and counseling individuals, and usually takes place within schools, health departments, community groups, and other health care systems.

In contrast, coalitions attempt to alleviate community problems by organizing the community to bring about change (Table 2-1 lists the ben-

efits associated with a community organizing approach). The general focus of community organizing is on changing a system, rules, social norms,
or laws, in order to ultimately change the legality and social acceptability
of behaviors. The venue for community organizing is in the policy arena,
and often involves community elected officials, businesses, community
groups, media, and local and state legislature. Community organizing is
an ongoing process that involves identifying the many facets of a problem
in a community and implementing a comprehensive plan to address the
issue through established community channels and systems.

STEPS TO COALITION BUILDING

Steps for building a coalition, as outlined in Table 2-2, are based on the
experiences of successful tobacco reduction coalitions in Michigan. This
list provides guidance on how to proceed with developing a coalition.

Analyzing the Issue

The first step in forming a coalition is to analyze the issue or problem in the
community. This can be accomplished by identifying and studying resource
documents and collecting data (both local and state) relative to the issue.
Many local health departments have conducted in-depth analyses, surveys,
focus groups and community assessments of health-related issues. These
data are available for public use. State, university, and state health department libraries have excellent resources including books, journals, and other
documents. Many health-related statistics are available through state vital
statistics offices, state agencies, community-based organizations, and community and state Internet sites. Also, centers for health promotion and
chronic disease prevention at state health departments often offer free resources, statistics, and consultation on health-related issues.

Table 2-1. Benefits of a Community Organizing Approach

- The potential to affect large numbers of people.
- Most interventions have a lasting impact.
- Creating a widespread public awareness of the issue.
- Creating public support for changes.
- Media interest in covering the issue and proposed changes.
- Increasing local policy maker's involvement and support.
- Reducing the social acceptability of health risk behaviors.
- Changing in community norms/standards.

Table 2-2. Steps for Building an Effective Coalition

1. Analyze the issue or problem on which the coalition will focus.
2. Create an awareness of the issue. (ongoing)
3. Host a coalition planning meeting, and invite key community members.
4. Recruit coalition members. (ongoing)
5. Elect coalition leadership.
6. Orient coalition members regarding the issue. (ongoing)
7. Develop the coalition's mission, goals, and objectives.
8. Develop strategic plans and programs.
9. Identify resources and funding needed to carry out strategies.
10. Break strategies down into tasks and decide who is responsible for each task.
11. Train coalition members in how to carryout the strategies.
12. Implement coalition strategies.
13. Involve local media in the coalition's efforts. (ongoing)
14. Evaluate coalition efforts relative to its mission, goals, and objectives and revise as needed. (ongoing)
15. Publicly recognize the efforts of the coalition membership. (ongoing)
16. Plan periodic appreciation events for active coalition membership. (ongoing)

Creating Awareness

It is essential to create public awareness of an issue in order to (1) raise public concern and support for the coalition and its strategies, (2) recruit coalition members, and (3) obtain funds for the coalition.

Creating public awareness can be accomplished by providing information on the issue to the local media including newspapers, radio, and television. A relationship with the media can be established by calling and introducing one's self to local reporters, newspaper editors, and other media personnel. Media networking may help in maximizing media coverage on the issue and increase the likelihood of becoming a future resource for the media (see Chapter 7, "Marketing and Public Relations," Chapter 8, "Media Advocacy," and Chapter 10, "Media and Advocacy Tools" for further skills related to working with media). Providing presentations to community groups and local officials on an issue and how it impacts community members can also create awareness, garner support for coalition development, and secure funding. It is important to remember that promoting community awareness of an issue is an ongoing process.

Some coalitions emerge because public awareness and concern about an issue already exists and funding is made available to help alleviate the problem. The legislature often will designate funding to allow for community prevention and control efforts on specific issues such as violence, tobacco, and diabetes.

Coalition Planning

Coalition planning can be conducted in different ways. It is recommended, however, that an initial planning meeting be organized. Local voluntary agencies (such as the American Heart Association or American Lung Association) and at least one elected official should be invited. The purpose of this meeting is to discuss the feasibility of developing a coalition. The following should be addressed in the planning meeting:[1]

- *Establishing a coalition.* Is it worth the effort? Are there other established human service coalitions or groups that might consider either broadening their interests to include the issue or establishing a subcommittee that would, in essence, become a coalition in itself? Some effective community coalitions are actually subcommittees of established broader human service collaborating bodies.

- *Brainstorming who else should be invited to join the coalition.* Potential coalition members should be identified using phone books, local government listings and human service agency, business, school, and other community directories. Agencies and other groups that currently focus their efforts on the same issue as the one for the proposed coalition should be included in the list of potential members. Parent groups, local voluntary associations, religious associations, youth groups, personal acquaintances, representatives of the target population(s), and representatives of the media should also be recruited. A coalition with a membership that reflects the diversity of the community is more likely to be successful.

- *Choosing a date, time, and place for the first coalition meeting.* The initial meeting should be scheduled at least one month in advance in order to reduce scheduling conflicts. If possible, this meeting should coincide with another meeting at which some of the potential members are likely to be in attendance (e.g., a human service coordinating council meeting). The best way(s) for inviting potential members (i.e., phone, mail, media, or personal visits) needs to be determined. Follow-up phone calls may increase the number of people who attend the first meeting.

- *Deciding who should lead the coalition.* An agency or individual needs to be identified who will continue taking the responsibility for initially leading the coalition effort. After the coalition is well established and, perhaps, some funding has been secured for the group, leadership should be elected.

- *Developing an agenda for the first coalition meeting.* The first coalition meeting is crucial. Individuals will likely decide at the first meeting if they will to become a member of the coalition or if their time could be better spent. The agenda should include an overview of the issue, coalition mission and goals, task force formation, meeting dates and times, and time for networking.

- *Contacting the media.* Someone with prior experience dealing with the media, or someone who is well versed on the issue and coalition plans, should be selected to contact the media regarding the establishment of the coalition. Press releases should be developed and distributed prior to the first coalition meeting.

- *Locating funding for the coalition.* A plan for securing funding needs to be developed. Potential funding sources include membership dues, grants, monetary donations, and in-kind contributions (e.g., postage, meeting rooms, food, office supplies, and secretarial time) from members. Attendees at the initial meeting should explore all potential funding sources that may exist in their professional and personal networks.

Membership Recruitment

Turnover of coalition members, new people arriving in the community, changing needs, and new ideas for including groups and individuals in the coalition, make the membership recruitment process a constant. Persuading people to join the coalition and give up their time and energy will take some effort, especially because potential members already participate in other committees and coalitions.

Some coalitions have had great success recruiting members by organizing membership drives. Successful approaches have included (1) marketing the coalition by providing information at community events, (2) placing ads in local newspapers, (3) requesting that businesses and human service organizations appoint a person to represent their organization on the coalition, (4) presenting information to religious groups and community associations about the issue and coalition plans to alleviate the problem, (5) appealing to area schools for students who are looking for community service opportunities, (6) requesting time on PTA/PTO agendas, and (7) approaching environmental groups for assistance on projects.

Personal contacts are generally more successful in recruiting members than mass mailings. Individuals who attend the coalition planning meeting should be able to assist with personal recruitment. Members can also be recruited through invitation letters from top administrators of lead organizations involved in the coalition planning group. Each organization that receives an invitation should be asked to appoint a representative to the coalition. Often a follow-up phone call is needed to establish which individuals have volunteered or been chosen to represent the various organizations.

Local chapters of associations related to the issue will likely wish to participate in the coalition. For example, with a tobacco coalition, relative organizations include the American Heart Association, American Lung Association, and American Cancer Society. Staff and volunteers associated with these organizations are dedicated to improving the health of their community and may be interested in serving on relevant coalitions.

Local policy makers and other influential individuals in the local community (e.g., local celebrities) may be interested in membership because of their commitment to the community and its potential to provide personal recognition and visibility. It is important to have a balance, however, between the "doers" and those lending their names and voices to the effort.

It is highly recommended that coalitions enlist support of volunteers interested in providing community service. Volunteers can often be located through a local volunteer action center, university or community college, high school, or voluntary association.

Members need to be actively recruited from all segments of the community (e.g., public and private, rich and poor, young and old). In doing so, sensitivity to cultural norms, values, and beliefs will be manifested in the coalition. Representatives from minority groups need to be included to ensure that action plans are suitable for diverse populations. In addition, individuals who either directly or indirectly suffer from disease or hardship relative to the issue should be encouraged to join, as they can provide an excellent source for understanding the issue better.

Offering potential members something in return for participating can be helpful in recruiting new members. For example, a certain organization may need assistance with media training or contacts so they can attract greater attention to their cause. Someone with media experience from the coalition could assist them in that area in return for their commitment to work on a specific coalition project.[3]

Another segment of the population from which to recruit members are youth. Organized youth groups such as 4-H Clubs, church groups, peer-to-peer counselors, local chapters of Students Taking A New Direction (STAND) and Students Against Drunk Driving (SADD), environmental youth clubs, and youth athletic clubs may be interested in joining the coalition or supporting specific coalition projects. Existing youth groups may be willing to adapt their mission statements to include the coalition issue. For example, a local youth group such as SADD could be asked to consider including other drugs, such as tobacco, in their mission and to work on specific tobacco coalition projects. Youth groups may welcome specific suggestions for activities.

No matter which segment of the population is being recruited for the coalition, personal motivation is a key factor to be considered. Generally, individuals will participate in coalitions because of their commitment to alleviating the problem. Other members participate because they gain a sense of satisfaction from volunteering and working with other professionals. Also, becoming active in a coalition can assist individuals in overcoming the sense of powerlessness that can discourage even the most committed advocates. It has been found that individuals are motivated to become members of coalitions based on the need to:[4]

- Fulfill a shared interest.

- Improve community services and the health of community members.

- Share resources, including money, staff, and materials that are in short supply.

- Be visible in the community and demonstrate civic responsibility.

Marketing efforts that consider why potential members might be motivated to join their coalition will likely enjoy much recruiting success.

Coalition Leadership

Capable leadership is integral to the success of a coalition. Leadership can be elected or appointed, formal or informal. Often the key to coalition leadership is the ability to delegate tasks to the membership, negotiate when differences of opinion arise, and communicate openly and effectively with the membership and the community.

Coalition leaders should know how to motivate members, but not push them too far. It is important for leaders to (1) be giving of time and expertise, (2) share credit for successes, (3) concentrate on coalition strengths rather than weaknesses, (4) know members well enough to be able to determine who can be counted on for extra support, (5) realize that coalition members' time is equally important, and (6) realize that community needs are great in many areas.[3] Coalition leadership generally consists of two positions: (1) Coalition Chairperson and (2) Coalition Coordinator.

Coalition Chairperson

Many coalitions opt to elect a chairperson for a one- or two-year period. The chairperson's responsibilities include leading meetings, public speaking, media relations, and directing projects. It is essential that the chairperson works closely with the coalition coordinator on tasks such as:[1]

- Setting meeting agendas.

- Ensuring that each meeting is well-organized.

- Encouraging member discussion and input.

- Delegating responsibilities to members.

- Bringing the coalition to consensus on issues.

- Conducting follow-up with members.

- Recruiting and recognizing membership.

- Appointing a media spokesperson.

- Dealing with difficult people and personalities.

- Setting up training for members.

Coalition Coordinator

The coalition coordinator, a job which can often be demanding and time consuming, is integral to the success of a coalition. Different from the coalition chairperson, the coordinator often works behind the scenes to organize the meetings, complete all necessary paperwork, recruit members, organize member orientation/training, and coordinate membership recognition. The success of a coalition often hinges on the coordinator's energy, commitment, persistence, and credibility. Frequent coordinator turnover has proven to be detrimental to the success of many coalitions.

The lead agency of the coalition generally is responsible for selecting or hiring the coalition coordinator. This individual should not be the same person who is elected to serve as coalition chair, but rather someone who was integral in the initial formation of the coalition. A health educator with community organizing interests and experience would be a natural fit for the coalition coordinator role.

Strategic Planning

After the coalition has been formed, its mission statement, goals, objectives, and strategies need to be developed. Coalitions often start by formulating the mission statement, which is usually one to three sentences describing what the coalition hopes to achieve, how it plans to accomplish goals, and for whose benefit the coalition exists. A sample mission statement might read: "The Apple County Cardiovascular Disease Prevention Coalition seeks to reduce the incidence of cardiovascular disease in Apple County Residents through networking, education, and advocacy efforts."

The coalition should also develop short- and long-term goals, which are generally non-measurable, broad statements of purpose. For each goal, objectives (which are short range, specific outcomes of a program or project) should be written. Objectives can be either process oriented (i.e., outlining who will perform the activity, what exactly will be done, and when the activity will take place) or outcome based (i.e., providing quantifiable, measurable courses of action that can be evaluated).

In the initial stages of coalition formation, a membership survey should be administered that identifies areas of interest and expertise, resources members can lend to the coalition efforts, and preference for meeting times and places. Results of the survey will identify strengths and interests that will aide in developing a formal structure consisting of a mission statement, goals and objectives, and strategies. Adapting mission statements and ideas for successful strategies from other community coalitions will help in avoiding "reinventing the wheel." Talking to health professionals from other areas, searching the Internet, and reviewing other health publications, may help locate other coalitions that are working on similar issues. Networking will likely provide valuable ideas and help save time and energy.

Strategic plans can help focus a coalition's limited resources and time on developing strategies to impact outcomes. Strategies for achieving coalition objectives should be (1) realistic and built on the experience of others, (2) flexible and take into account that obstacles can occur, (3) respectful of organizational cultures, and (4) designed to enhance coalition unity. Also, effective strategies are educational and take into account that people learn as much from the process as from the end result.[5] Example strategies include (1) organizing a cardiovascular disease conference for area physicians and nurses that focuses on developing a standard system for counseling patients on heart disease risk reduction, and (2) conducting a media event (e.g., press conference) to highlight the success of the community mall walking project in lowering the blood pressure rates and body fat ratios of participants. Strategies are often implemented by subcommittees of the coalition. This may mean that there are several ongoing strategies being implemented by the coalition at the same time.

In the beginning, it is recommended that coalitions pursue strategies that are both noncontroversial and "easy wins." These strategies could include booths at community events to promote community awareness about an issue, youth poster contests in the schools to promote a theme in the community, and providing awards to individuals and businesses that have made an impact on the problem on which the coalition is focusing. Small successes are very important to build the confidence and unity of the membership. There is no guarantee, however, that even the best planned strategy will be successful. As coalitions develop experience, members will learn from their mistakes and successes, resulting in easier and more effective strategizing.[5]

Funding

Funding to support coalition efforts can come from numerous sources including grants, in-kind donations from members, donations from community or civic groups, donations from the business sector, membership dues, and fund-raising events.

Grants are often available through state and federal agencies, private foundations, local community agencies, and businesses. They usually have very specific guidelines for activities, may involve significant reporting requirements and other paperwork, and come with certain restrictions on how the money can and cannot be spent, which may force a coalition to narrow or broaden its focus in order to qualify. Before applying for a grant, a coalition needs to consider whether the benefits of receiving a grant outweigh the responsibilities, requirements, and restrictions.

Effective coalitions are usually successful at seeking and securing donations from local businesses and community organizations. This is often due to a coalition's visibility in the community and public awareness of its accomplishments. Many businesses and community groups look for opportunities to be associated with something positive happening in their community and may give money in exchange for their business' name being listed as a sponsor of coalition materials or projects. Businesses that often contribute services to the coalition in exchange for recognition include printers, office supply stores, public relation firms, hospitals and other health care organizations, and restaurants. Community groups that would be likely to contribute funds to community coalition efforts include service groups such as the Lion's Club, Rotary Club, Zonta Club, and Junior League. Requests for funding involve delegating specific coalition members to make phone calls, attend meetings and conduct presentations about the coalition, its goals, and needs for financial assistance.

Membership dues often involve an annual set fee from each individual member and organization. Dues should be no more than needed to cover expenses. Because membership fees may discourage some individuals from participating, instituting dues should be used with caution.

Fund-raisers (e.g., bake sales and car washes) can be very time consuming and could lead the coalition away from its original mission. They generally have a low rate of return on time invested and should, therefore, be used only when necessary.

Generally, coalitions do not need vast amounts of funding to be effective. Sometimes a large coalition budget can cause problems such as focusing too much time and energy encumbering funds, debating how to spend the money, and paying bills. If one agency contributes most of the funds for the coalition (through a grant or other source), contributions from other member organizations may decrease, which could ultimately diminish team work, involvement, and support from other members. In addition, if one agency contributes the bulk of the funding for the coalition, it may feel the need to control the coalition agenda. A lack of shared input can be detrimental to the development of the coalition as a true partnership. Coalitions that involve a broad spectrum of people from the community as equal partners are most successful at building support and locating funding sources within their communities.

CHARACTERISTICS OF A SUCCESSFUL COALITION

Coalitions are established for many different reasons and may focus on a variety of issues. Regardless of the focus, there are a number of common factors that have been found to contribute to the success of a coalition (see Table 2-3).[6] In contrast, factors that *have not* been found to impact the success of a coalition include the total number of coalition members, the total number and regularity of coalition meetings, and the existence of coalition subcommittees. Process oriented issues, like those listed in Table 2-3, rather than coalition structure, tend to have a greater influence on the success of the coalition.

Successful coalitions often engage coalition members by providing them with tasks in their area of interest or expertise. Working on issues in which members are interested increases member ownership and commitment. The key is to get to know each of the members personally and to find common interests that will benefit individual members and the coalition. Paying tribute to members for their efforts in the coalition is important. Through public and personal recognition, members feel their efforts are worthwhile and appreciated. Activities for member recognition could include hosting a recognition breakfast, sending letters of appreciation to members and their supervisors at work, publishing a program newsletter that includes highlights of members' involvement, presenting certificates of service, and soliciting area businesses to provide complimentary tickets for community events.[1]

Coalitions are often successful when they work through established community events rather than spending time initiating new ones. For example, many communities have avenues in place such as the American Heart Association's *Great American Smokeout*, community health fairs, and

Table 2-3. Characteristics of Successful Coalitions

- Continuity of coalition staff, in particular the coordinator position.
- Diversity of groups and individuals involved.
- Agreement on a common unifying purpose.
- Community leaders support the coalition and its efforts.
- Active involvement of community volunteer agencies.
- Common vocabulary among coalition members.
- Frequent and ongoing training for coalition members.
- Needs of coalition members are met in some way.
- Active involvement of members in developing coalition goals, objectives, and strategies.
- Productive coalition meetingsæthe group does not meet just to talk.
- Core group of active members assist in implementing strategies.
- Consensus is reached on issues instead of voting.
- Ownership of the problem by coalition members and community.
- Development of a strategic action plan versus a "project-by-project" approach.
- High level of trust and reciprocity among members.
- Active involvement by local media.
- Large problems are broken down into smaller, solvable pieces.

free hospital breast cancer screenings. By capitalizing on these events, coalitions can contribute with very little funding.

STRATEGIES FOR OVERCOMING BARRIERS

All coalitions face problems or barriers that hinder its ability to achieve goals and objectives. These problems could seriously impact the effectiveness of the coalition and set back community efforts to address the issue. Common problems that coalitions face are listed in Table 2-4. The following suggestions can assist coalitions in avoiding barriers known to impede success:[5]

- Deal with differences of opinion by trying to compromise and come to a consensus on issues. Angry members can undermine the coalition in the community. If necessary, try to deal with angry members in private.

- Ensure membership recognition and retention are high priorities.

- Politely ask groups that remain uncertain and uncommitted to the cause to leave the coalition.

- Obtain a high level of commitment from top administrators of lead organizations and ensure that their commitment is communicated regularly to the coalition and the general public.

- Seek representation on, or periodically communicate with, all other major community coalitions and committees.

- Clearly define the coalition mission and member responsibilities.

- Watch out for hidden agendas.

- Do not let the major contributors to the coalition control the agenda. Domination might deprive other groups of their sense of equal participation. Consider setting a membership fee for all members.

- Utilize humor with the coalition when appropriate. Do not become weighed down by the seriousness of the issue.

- Ensure coalition membership represents a large variety of people and organizations.

Delegating tasks and reducing conflict are skills that coalition leaders must have in order for the coalition to function smoothly. Many of the barriers listed in Table 2-4 can be eliminated by implementing effective use of delegation and conflict resolution skills.

Delegating Tasks

Delegation is the process of transferring to coalition members (1) responsibility—the obligation to carry out an assignment, (2) authority—the power necessary to assure the end result is achieved, and (3) accountability—the responsibility for results. Delegation is important because the coalition staff cannot, and should not, do all of the coalition work. It promotes a sense of ownership for the coalition among its members—the coalition is not one agency's initiative but a shared initiative among all members. Engaging many members in coalition efforts will have more impact than utilizing the energy of only one or two people.

In order to effectively delegate tasks, the goals for the coalition and its projects should be clearly stated. Job descriptions should be developed for coalition member duties, and volunteer workers should be actively recruited and trained in skills needed to accomplish coalition objectives. Leaders must be able to release control of the process and details associated with coalition activities, and encourage ownership and mutual input on expected outcomes, strategies, and the like. Lastly, an environment that fosters initiative and rewards results should be cultivated.[7] In contrast, cer-

Table 2-4. Common Problems that Coalitions Experience

- Too many planners and not enough "doers."
- Difficulty engaging local policy makers in the cause.
- Not enough high-level administrative support from the coalition organizations to implement coalition strategies.
- Difficulty coming to a consensus about what should be done.
- Difficulty going beyond planning strategies.
- Membership burnout and turnover.
- Lack of training among coalition members.
- Not enough coordinator time allocated to adequately staff the coalition.

tain characteristics are likely to hinder the coalition leader's successful delegation of tasks (see Table 2-5).

Reducing Conflict

Conflict is normal and inevitable when working with people who are trying to agree upon and achieve mutual goals. Conflicts are frequently the basis for defensiveness, reduced communication, and the termination of relationships among members of a group. Sources of conflict include (1)

Table 2-5. Characteristics that Hinder Task Delegation

- Unclear goals and objectives.
- Attitude of "doer"ædoing things by self versus working with others to accomplish tasks.
- "I can do it better and faster" syndrome.
- A desire to engage in enjoyable tasks alone.
- Unwillingness to transfer the responsibility and authority to untrained or inexperienced staff.
- Insecurities.
- Insufficiently organized to provide directives and ensure they are carried through.
- Unwillingness to let someone else determine the method and details.
- Perfectionism.
- Aversion to risk.
- Performing several tasks instead of concentrating on management of the coalition.
- Organizational instability.
- Lack of resources.
- Poorly defined accountability.

differences in values and goals; (2) allocation of scarce resources like money, facilities, and time; (3) perceived threats to autonomy, rights, or identity; and (4) differences in relation to how desired ends should be achieved.

If not addressed and minimized, conflict can cripple a coalition. Conflict can, however, be resolved in constructive ways that will likely enhance future collaboration and creativity. Table 2-6 contains suggestions that can help reduce conflict within coalitions.[1]

EVALUATING COALITION SUCCESS

Evaluation is an important part of developing and maintaining a coalition. It is usually difficult, however, to link coalition efforts to empirical end points because coalitions often work on long-term projects (e.g., changing community policies) that may ultimately affect personal behaviors. A long period of time may lapse before the behavior change takes place and can be surveyed or recorded. For instance, it is difficult in the short term to measure if a coalition project designed for promoting parents to quit smoking impacts whether children will start to smoke. Evaluation is also difficult because data needed to evaluate coalition efforts are usually not collected. Funding is usually spent on intervention rather than evaluation efforts, making it difficult to evaluate coalition effectiveness.

Table 2-6. Strategies for Reducing Conflict

- Rotate leadership at least every two years to address conflict arising out of the sharing of power.
- Separate individuals from the problem. Let individuals express their differences and work together to resolve them.
- Use formal group process techniques to address conflict arising from lack of full participation in meetings or from the over participation by some.
- Distribute information relative to the coalition or its issue as it becomes available.
- Rotate meeting sites to reduce "turf" battles.
- Do not allow "either-or" thinking. Require that dissenting parties generate a third alternative to "my way" or "your way."
- Rule out the use of "you" messages and personal accusations. Instruct members to suggest a joint effort to locate the source of the problem.
- Change seating arrangements. Creatively seat parties next to (as opposed to across from) each other. Rotate seating to promote or reduce communication.
- Search for areas of agreement and trust.
- Take a break from the topic until emotions have cooled.

Given these difficulties, there are a number of different types of evaluation that may be appropriate for coalitions:[7]

- *Process evaluation.* Documenting what was done and how many people were reached by coalition interventions. With this form of evaluation, record keeping of coalition efforts is important. An annual report, highlighting the coalition accomplishments and numbers of people served, can be used to report process results.

- *Impact evaluation.* Documenting accomplishments of specific objectives. This type of evaluation determines the extent to which the coalition efforts were effective. Impact evaluation results can be helpful for raising funds for additional coalition activities.

- *Outcome evaluation.* Measuring change in prevalence rates. This is a long-term evaluation that involves measuring the effect coalition efforts have had on key community indicators. Due to the inability to control extraneous variables, however, it is difficult to accurately determine the long-term effect of coalition efforts.

Coalitions should conduct regular evaluation in order to justify refunding, gain additional support, demonstrate the effectiveness of various programs, and provide a basis for future planning.[6]

EXPECTED OUTCOMES

A number of outcomes associated with community coalition efforts will occur. Some of the more important include the following:

- *Partnerships and relationships are established among community agencies, individuals, and influential people.* These relationships are developed through networking and collaboration and may be useful in focusing on other community issues in the future.

- *Relationships with the media develop.* As coalition staff and members strive to accomplish their goals, they probably will have (1) had frequent contact with reporters, (2) written letters to the editor of local papers, and (3) spoken on local radio or television. A relationship is built in which the coalition and members become recognized by the media as experts on the issue. As a result, the media will often take the initiative to contact someone from the coalition the next time the issue is referenced.

- *Public awareness is raised and community and social change is initiated.* Creating community awareness of an issue often leads to changes in individual beliefs and personal habits, as well as public policy. Many times changes in public policy proceed changes in personal habits. For example, businesses that establish smoke-free policies may influence employees to quit smoking.

- *Legislators and local policy makers become aware of the coalition and its potential influence.* Coalitions tend to be highly visible in communities and can easily draw the attention and interest of legislators and local policy makers. These individuals are interested in having their names associated with initiatives that lead to positive changes in their communities.

- *Coalition members and community members are empowered from their experiences.* The process of implementing coalition strategies tends to create a sense of accomplishment and a "can do" and "can make a difference" attitude with coalition members, target audiences, and the community as a whole.

- *Each person, or organization, within a coalition becomes part of a greater whole.* They now speak to the problem with a combined power and a unified voice.[7] This combined power is much greater than what each organization can accomplish alone. Issues become solvable because individuals and agencies in the community begin to talk with each other and take ownership for the community problem.

- *Development of a community standard of what is and is not acceptable.* A coalition that addresses an issue and creates awareness of the risks, benefits, and possible solutions related to an issue, can promote changing a community norm of what is and is not acceptable. Coalition efforts become a process of setting the community standard of beliefs and behavior.

CONCLUSION

Coalition building can be challenging, time consuming, and frustrating. Most often, however, the benefits far outweigh these drawbacks. Coalition building can benefit both communities and individual health professionals. As presented in this chapter, community benefits are numerous, including the ultimate reduction of the community health problem or issue. For health educators, serving on coalitions can expand professional networks, enhance personal knowledge and experiences in community organizing, and assist in achieving professional goals associated with health promotion and disease prevention.

References

1. Whitt, M. (1993). *Fighting tobacco: A coalition approach to improving your community's health.* Lansing, MI: Michigan Department of Public Health.

2. McLeroy, K., Kegler, M., Steckler, A., Burdine, J., & Wisotzky, M. (1994). Community coalitions for health promotion: Summary and further reflections. *Health Education Research, 9*(1), 1-11.

3. Stop Teenage Addiction to Tobacco. (1992). *Community organizers' manual* (pp. 35-36). Springfield, MA: Author.

4. Minnesota Department of Health. (1988). *A guide for promoting health in Minnesota: A community approach.* St. Paul, MN: Author.

5. Pertschuk, M. (1988). Smoking or health: The coalition as giant killer. Keynote address to the Michigan Coalition on Smoking or Health Training Conference for Volunteers, March 18, Lansing, MI.

6. Merenda, D. (1986). *A practical guide to creating and managing school/community partnerships.* Alexandria, VA: National School Volunteer Program, Inc.

7. American Stop Smoking Intervention Study. (1991). *Orientation manual.* Washington DC: National Cancer Institute

Chapter 3

CONDUCTING FOCUS GROUPS

Lisa R. Rutherford, M.A., C.H.E.S.

Author's Comments: *Focus groups can be an excellent tool to use in community assessment, program planning, marketing, and evaluation. In nearly every health and human service field, and in nearly every community-based coalition, it seems that focus groups have taken root as part of the planning and assessment process. Having been involved with various focus group projects, I find this both exciting and a little unnerving all at the same time. It is exciting to see that more people, whose voices might otherwise have been silent, are increasingly being given the opportunity to have input when community planning takes place. It is gratifying to know that what people in the community think, feel, and believe is important and is starting to influence policy, decision making, and funding. As any focus group participant will most likely indicate, it is gratifying for them to know this, too.*

At the same time, I remain a bit skeptical when I hear that yet another focus group project has been conducted in the community. The skepticism is due to the fact that many agencies and coalitions run focus groups without a solid understanding of the process. When the process is not fully understood, focus groups might be used inappropriately, the project might not be properly planned, the focus groups may not be properly conducted, or the data analysis may be inaccurate. I strongly advise anyone who is planning to engage in a focus group project to learn the method as well as possible, so that such pitfalls can be avoided.

Before my first attempt at a focus group project, I engaged in hours of self-study and consultation with others who had experience in focus groups. While I learned a great deal before I started planning and conducting focus groups, I can honestly say that I learn more each time I am involved in a project. Not only do I learn about planning and conducting focus groups, I learn more about the people in the community.

INTRODUCTION

A focus group is a unique qualitative research technique used to gather information on opinions, perceptions, and ideas about a specified topic. This interview technique has made its way into social science research from marketing research, where the method has long been used to ascertain consumer opinions. A focus group approach may be used as the sole method of data gathering, but has particular strength when used in conjunction with other forms of qualitative data collection methods (e.g., key informant interviews, field observation) or to complement quantitative research methods (e.g., statistical data, survey findings).[1]

Focus groups may be used to assist in the initial design of surveys and questionnaires to be administered to larger populations. For example, a tri-county area substance abuse coalition in Michigan was preparing to administer a survey to sponsors of parent education programs to determine program availability related to the prevention of substance abuse in children. The original survey included questions pertaining to days of the week and times of day that parent education programs were offered, as well as geographic locations of the programs. After the initial survey was developed, it was clear that the survey did not assess program content, which would allow professionals to see the range of topics being offered in the area's parent education programs. There also were no questions geared toward assessment of information that parents felt were relevant to preventing substance abuse in their children, which could serve as an incentive for parents to attend programs.

The coalition decided these two elements were critical in determining availability of meaningful parent education programs, and decided to redesign the survey. This was accomplished by holding a series of focus groups with parents to determine (1) information parents were interested in learning about substance abuse prevention, (2) information parents thought was important to know about preventing substance abuse in children, and (3) parents' perceptions of the relationship between the parenting role and substance use in children. A series of focus groups were also conducted among a range of professionals (e.g. teachers, probate court staff, law enforcement, medical professionals) to determine their opinions on the same topics, but from their perspectives as professionals in specific fields. Data were then analyzed and used to develop a more comprehensive survey that assessed program content. This enabled the coalition to better determine if the programs being offered matched the community's interest and opinion of need relative to the subject.

Focus groups also may be chosen as a follow-up to primary methods of data collection, such as to enhance program outcome evaluation or to aid in the comprehension of poorly understood survey results.[1] For example, a local abstinence coalition implemented focus groups in a sample of seventh-grade students that received a coalition sponsored abstinence-based curriculum. The focus group approach was used to identify (1) the types of knowledge the students retained from the curriculum, (2) if the students practiced the skills taught in the curriculum, and (3) suggestions the students had for improving the curriculum. This allowed coalition members to determine if students were able to process the information taught in the curriculum and to understand "real-life" situations in which the students applied the learned knowledge and skills. The students' opinions helped the presenters fine tune the curriculum to better meet the needs and interests of the students and helped demonstrate the curriculum's value to coalition members.

There are many appropriate uses for focus groups in the health education and health planning fields. Information on attitudes and perceptions about health issues, programs, and prevention and intervention strategies, can be obtained from focus groups. They can be used to gather opinions on existing programs and services, to generate ideas for improving programs and services, or in developing new resources.

Typically, focus groups range in size from 8 to 12 participants. The participants generally are homogenous, having been selected because they have similar characteristics that relate to the topic of the focus group discussion.[2] A series of focus groups (usually at least two or three in a population group) surrounding the same topic are conducted to allow the researcher to discern patterns of thought and themes of importance to the participants. Focus group discussions are led by a moderator who possesses skills in group dynamics and interview techniques. The moderator follows a predetermined discussion guide containing open-ended questions developed around a defined topic. As with any data collection technique, the focus group method possesses certain strengths and limitations as a means of data collection (see Table 3-1).

FOCUS GROUP IMPLEMENTATION

Those who fail to plan, plan to fail. These words of wisdom are highly applicable when it comes to implementing focus groups. Successful implementation of focus group data collection depends greatly on the thoroughness of the planning that goes into the project.

Project Proposal

When planning a focus group project, the first step is to prepare a project plan, or proposal, and submit it to a funding source (e.g., a sponsoring agency, or a coalition) if funding or approval is needed to make the project a reality. The proposal identifies, at a minimum, (1) the rationale for proposing the use of focus groups as a means of data collection, (2) a description of focus group method including the method's strengths and limitations, (3) who will be using the results and how, (4) a time line, and (5) a budget. The proposal might also outline plans for participant recruitment,

Table 3-1. Strengths and Limitations of Focus Groups

Strengths

1. Large amounts of data from a group of individuals is obtained quickly and often at proportionately lower costs than under individual interview or survey methods.

2. The moderator can clarify responses and probe for further understanding of poorly understood responses.

3. Observation of nonverbal cues (body language, facial expressions, etc.) provide insight into spoken responses.

4. Information is obtained in the participants' own words, which can be powerful in understanding perceptions and ideas and in communicating results.

5. Focus groups can be used to obtain information from illiterate individuals.

Limitations

1. Participants are generally self-selected, and are usually not representative of a random sample of the population. Therefore, their opinions and perceptions may differ from nonparticipants, making generalizability of the results to the larger population limited.

2. Opinionated participants or poorly skilled moderators can influence the discussion and therefore bias the results.

3. One focus group is usually not adequate in determining themes or patterns in results because groups can vary widely from one to the next.

4. Transcription and data analysis can be time consuming.

data analysis and moderator selection (if outside moderators will be used), as these elements are generally the most time consuming and most costly aspects of the focus group technique.

The time line and budget are critical elements in any proposal, particularly if approval is required before the project can proceed. Various texts on the focus group technique, and practical experience, have shown there to be a wide degree of variation in both the estimated number of hours needed to complete the individual steps in the focus group design and in cost.

Recruitment

The most time-consuming step in the focus group approach is participant recruitment. It is always wise to allow for more time than originally planned for this task. Unlike other recruitment processes, focus group participant recruitment can be complex because people are asked to travel to a location *you* have selected, at a time *you* have selected, and to use two hours of their free time to discuss a topic *you* have selected. It is wise to start with a list of at least 30 to 40 potential participants for *each* focus group as many individuals who are contacted decline the invitation to participate.

Prior to contacting potential participants, a short screening questionnaire should be developed to allow recruiters to narrow the field to only those with the specific characteristics desired (see Figure 3-1). Any person assisting in the recruitment process should be provided with a written list of specific characteristic or demographic criteria and a copy of the screening script. After individuals have been determined as eligible, they should be provided with information about the focus group project, including who is funding and coordinating the project, the purpose of the study, how the results will be used and how confidentiality will be maintained. These specific items are contained within the screening script. Many people are skeptical about participating in focus groups—particularly if the topic is controversial—and a guarantee of confidentiality can be critical in getting individuals to agree to participate.

Participants for focus groups can be found from a number of sources. Asking members of community-based coalitions, service agencies, or key community leaders to suggest potential participants is one strategy commonly used. Anyone who is recommending participants should have a clear understanding as to what specific participant characteristics or demographics are desired. It will be a great help if those who recommend potential participants can make initial contact with the individual to determine their willingness or interest in participating. They should provide the names, addresses and phone numbers of only those individuals who agree to participate, or who might be interested but would like more information.

· Participants can also be generated from mailing or membership lists which might be made available through a number of resources such as professional or charitable organizations, community-based organizations, civic organizations, or newsletter mailing lists. Again, it is helpful if an individual within the organization or agency providing the list can randomly select individuals to be contacted to measure their interest and to receive permission to share their names, addresses, and phone numbers.

If the budget allows, random selection can be made from a purchased sample of telephone numbers. Cold calls to randomly selected numbers (e.g., every nth number) may take more time than using networks of contacts, but is an alternative way to randomly select participants. This method, however, limits the potential field of participants to only those who have telephones, and should be noted as a limitation in the final report.

Recruitment can also be made through face-to-face contact. For example, if participants who are consumers of a particular service (e.g., WIC, family planning) are needed, recruitment can be executed as individuals enter the agency—provided permission is granted from the appropriate supervisors and the appropriate personnel are made aware of the recruitment activity.

Figure 3-1. Sample Focus Group Recruitment Screening Script

Hello, my name is (*your name*) and I am calling on behalf of (*your organization or sponsoring agency*). I am recruiting participants for a small group discussion, called a focus group, in which we will be discussing the topic of (*name of topic*). Your name was given to us by (*name or organization*), who thought you might be interested in participating in this project. Do you have a few minutes right now to talk more about this project?

First, I need to ask a few questions to determine if you are eligible to participate in the focus group. This information will remain completely confidential and will not be linked to you in any way. The purpose of asking these questions is to simply make sure that the participants in the focus group match the needs of (*your organization or the sponsoring agency*).

(*Insert questions pertaining to specified characteristics here*)

Great! You are eligible to participate in the focus group. A focus group is a meeting of between 8 to 12 people. The group meets one time, and, in this case, will be discussing (*insert topic and, if preferred, a list of the major topic areas to be discussed from the discussion guideline*). You will not be asked to share any personal experiences, only your opinions and ideas.

The information that we find from the focus group will be put into a report for (*your organization or the sponsoring agency*). The report will be used to (*identify the purpose of the study, e.g., to plan for future health prevention programs or to evaluate the effectiveness of a provided service*). Your name will not be used in any report, nor will it be shared with anyone at any time. Whatever you say in the focus group can not be matched to you personally.

The meeting will be tape recorded so that we can have an accurate report written of what was discussed at the meeting. It is taped only to make certain that we do not misinterpret or leave out anything that was said. The tapes will be destroyed as soon as the report is written.

The focus group meeting will take between 1 1/2 to 2 hours. It is scheduled for (*time*) on (*date*) at (*location*). A free meal and child care will be provided. For your assistance, you will receive (*incentive*) upon completion of the focus group.

Does this sound like something in which you would be willing to participate?

Are you free at (*time*) on (*date*)?

Do you need child care? How many children do you have? What are their ages? (*If needed, provide information on child care arrangements here*).

Do you have transportation to the location? (*If no, provide details of transportation assistance here*).

Do you have any special dietary needs?

I will send you a letter to confirm everything that we have talked about today. Do you have an address at which you prefer to have this information sent?

If you have any questions, please contact (*name and address*). On behalf of (*your organization or the sponsoring agency*), I thank you for your assistance.

The use of advertisements for focus group recruitment is a practice that is discouraged largely because control can easily be lost over the number of participants and in the homogeneity of group members. It is important to limit the number of participants in a focus group to no more than 12. As group size increases, it becomes more difficult to guide discussion and several spontaneous "mini-discussions" can arise if members feel they are not able to share their opinions with the larger group.[2]

Using existing groups, such as service clubs or church groups, is also not widely practiced because members may not feel they can share their opinions and thoughts openly with people they know. Focus groups are sometimes used to gain opinions of people who are closely linked, such as residents of a housing complex or employees of an agency. In recruiting participants from existing groups, the fact that some or all participants were known to one another may influence individual responses, and should be considered during data analysis and in the reporting of the results.

After participants have been identified, confirmation letters should be sent that include the details of the focus group time and location, a map, and the incentive, if one is offered (see Figure 3-2). Also included should be the name, address, and phone number of a contact person to notify in case of cancellation or for further questions. The letter should be mailed 7 to 10 days in advance of the focus group meeting. A reminder phone call, placed to participants with telephones one to two days in advance of the focus group, may increase participation.

On average, initial recruitment calls take about 5 to 10 minutes per individual, giving a rough estimate of 6 to 12 calls per hour. This includes all contacts—some of those whom are contacted will decline to participate. It may be necessary to invite a few more individuals than are actually wanted in the focus group to accommodate for no-shows. Roughly 10% to 25% of confirmed participants will probably not show up for the focus group.[2]

Location

One of the easiest and often least expensive steps in the planning process is identifying a location to hold the focus groups. Many communities have meeting rooms that will accommodate small discussion groups. The selected location should be easily accessible for participants, barrier free, quiet, and free from outside noise or distraction. The moderator and all participants should be able to see one another. A location should be selected that will be viewed as a comfortable, neutral setting to participants. Religious institutions, hospitals, and health and human service agencies, in particular, may conjure up uncomfortable feelings for participants. Public libraries, schools, and community centers are usually better choices. Many meeting rooms can be used free of charge. If a fee is involved, it might help to speak with a manager or director at the location about the focus group project. Many times fees are waived in the interest of aiding a worthy cause.

Moderators

Another important step in preparation for the focus group is to determine who will moderate the discussions and who will assist the moderator as recorder. Moderator selection is based on factors such as experience with group dynamics, the ability to tactfully bring the discussion back on track when it begins to lose focus, and an ability to probe for further under-standing without making participants feel put on-the-spot. The moderator must have the ability to gently encourage quieter members to share and to delicately address members who dominate the discussion. Some knowl-edge of the subject area is desirable and can be of great value in spontane-ously developing probing questions. Moderators must take caution and make no leading remarks nor offer personal opinions, both of which can inhibit participants from freely expressing their thoughts and opinions.

Identification with the participants in terms of demographic charac-teristics is often advantageous in raising comfort and trust levels among participants, particularly in terms of racial or ethnic backgrounds. Mod-erators who are members of the same racial or ethnic group as the partici-pants are more likely to recognize and respect even the most subtle cul-tural nuances in the group process. Bilingual and, preferably, bicultural moderators and assistant moderators for foreign language speaking groups are a necessity. Using a translator to translate between languages during the focus group discussion causes chaos and frustration for both the mod-erator and the participants, and complicates the already delicate task of analysis. All participants within a focus group need to speak the same lan-guage so that each member can fully participate in the discussion.

In conducting focus groups with participants of various cultural back-grounds, cultural influences on the group process should be considered. For instance, in some cultures, female members may tend to defer to male members for appropriate responses, or younger members may wait for elder members to respond first. If the discussion will involve sensitive or potentially controversial topics, such as sexuality issues or contraception, consideration needs to be given as to the composition of group members. These factors, as well as the fact that some meaning may be lost in transla-tion between languages, should be taken into consideration during data analysis and presented in the final report.

The assistant moderator is responsible for managing many of the details surrounding the actual focus group execution, such as arranging the room prior to the participants' arrival, keeping track of time for the

Figure 3-2. Sample Confirmation Letter

(*name and address*)

On (*date*), you spoke with a representative from (*name of the organization*) about participating in a focus group on the topic of (*name of topic*). The focus group is part of a project being organized by the (*name of the organization*) for the purpose of (*include information on purpose of the study*).

The focus group in which you agreed to participate will meet at the following time and place:

> **Date:**
> **Time:**
> **Location:**
> **Address:**

(*include information about directions, transportation details, child care details, and confirmation of special dietary needs, if appropriate*)

It is important that you are on time for this focus group meeting. It is also important that you plan on staying for the full duration. There will be a meal for you (*after/before*) the focus group meeting. You are encouraged to arrive 15 to 30 minutes early, if possible, so you can meet your fellow group members.

A report will be written about the focus group meeting. In order to write an accurate report, we will be tape-recording the meeting. We do, however, understand your right to privacy, and your name will not be used in any report or in any record of the focus group project.

Once again, thank you for agreeing to be a part of the focus group. In order to show our gratitude for your participation, you will receive (*incentive*) at the end of the focus group meeting.

Please feel free to contact (*name, phone number, address*) if you have any questions, or if you will be unable to participate in the focus group.

Sincerely,

(*name and address*)

---

moderator so that key questions are covered in the time allotted, verifying that all tapes used for recording are properly labeled, and making any tape changes necessary during the discussion. The assistant also has the responsibility of keeping detailed notes on nonverbal signals, environmental factors, and other circumstances that may improve data analysis. Placing numbered cardboard nameplates in front of each seat, asking participants to write their first names only next to the number as they arrive and take a seat, will enable the assistant to make notes of speaker numbers and a few key words from their dialogue during the discussion. This will ease speaker identification during transcription while still protecting confidentiality.

Immediately following the focus group session, the moderator and assistant moderator should share their overall impressions about the session and identify what each saw as major themes and important ideas in the discussion. This information is either taped or written down as soon as possible after the focus group session and submitted for use as part of the overall data analysis.

Moderators and assistant moderators may come from within or outside of the sponsoring agency, depending on the skills and time availability of staff. In contracting for these services, training is essential to ensure the moderators thoroughly understand the focus group process. The moderators' training should cover details of the particular focus group research in which they are participating, including safeguards necessary to maintain participant confidentiality. Expected outcomes of the project and how results will be used should be thoroughly explained. Moderators will need a contact person for any questions they or participants may have that are unable to be answered. Contractual moderators are typically compensated for training, travel and preparation time, and mileage, as well as for conducting the focus group. Moderators may be offered a flat rate to cover all these expenses as opposed to an hourly rate. The actual rate of compensation will depend on moderator skill level, current wage ranges, and the total budget available for the focus group project.

Discussion Guide

The discussion guide outlines the questions the moderator will use in facilitating the focus group. This guide typically contains open-ended questions in three or four related topic areas, moving from more general ideas and concepts to those that are more specific.[2] Within each topic area, there are usually two to four essential questions to be asked of the participants. Each of the main questions may be accompanied by suggested probes to foster the depth of the discussion, or to encourage responses from participants. Skilled moderators, who are familiar with the topic of discussion, may spontaneously develop their own probing questions during the focus group if further clarification of responses is needed.

The discussion guide may also include a scripted introduction to the focus group concept and the purpose of the focus group at hand for the benefit of participants. This type of introduction can help participants understand the nature of the focus group technique, why they have been selected as participants, and how the data will be used. The inclusion of an introductory script can be helpful if the moderator is not directly involved with the project development and, therefore, might need assistance in accurately explaining the purpose of the study and the use of the focus group results.

The amount of time needed to develop the discussion guide depends on various factors. This step moves much quicker if only one or two people have the responsibility to develop and approve the guide. Sometimes, however, this may not be the case. A committee, for example, may want the full membership involved in the development and approval of the guide. Or, perhaps, the guide must go through an internal chain of command for review by committee members or the sponsoring organization. In these cases, more time will be needed to call the necessary individuals together to develop the draft, for all appropriate persons to review and comment on the guide, and for revising the draft and possibly going through a final review and approval process. Again, the newer the writer of the discussion guide to the focus group technique, the longer it may take to develop a set of clear and concise, jargon-free, questions that will yield the type of data needed for the study. A safe estimate for the time needed to develop the discussion guide is six to eight hours, if three or fewer people are involved.

Recording Equipment

Taping the focus group will increase the likelihood of an accurate analysis. While some prefer videotaping to ease in the recall of nonverbal cues and in speaker identification, audiotaping is also completely acceptable. Videotaping requires special room setup and possibly use of multiple cameras so that every participant is captured on film. The presence of videotaping equipment may raise the level of discomfort with some members and could inhibit discussion, as it offers less anonymity than audiotaping.2

Whichever method is chosen, the equipment needs to be tested well in advance of the focus group and just prior to participants' expected arrival time. It is essential to bring backup recording equipment, extra tapes and batteries, and extension cords. Boom-boxes and hand-held tape recorders are not the best choices for taping group discussions. Many business and office supply companies carry recording equipment especially designed for recording group discussions. This type of equipment can be expensive and difficult to justify buying for a onetime focus group project. Some companies rent equipment at reasonable rates on a daily, weekly, or monthly basis.

Another possibility for transcribing the discussion is to hire a court reporter. While the cost for hiring a court reporter to attend several focus groups may be much higher than using recording equipment, it can save time and money in the end because the tape will not have to be transcribed by another party, which can take several hours for one focus group discussion. The court reporter must have the capability of putting the transcript on a computer diskette if a computer software-based analysis of all focus group discussions is planned.

Transcription and Analysis

A common method for analysis of focus groups is to analyze a verbatim transcript of the discussion made from audiotapes. The transcriber should indicate pauses, tears, laughter, and other relevant verbal cues that are evident on the tape. Inaudible dialogue should also be referenced in the transcript by simply stating "inaudible statements" or another similar phrase. Any names or other personal identifiers used in personal stories should be removed by the transcriber and noted in the transcript.[3] For example, if a participant references an individual by name, the name should be removed and replaced with a nonspecific pronoun or title e.g., "Dr. X" instead of "Dr. Smith," or "my brother (name excluded)" instead of "my brother, Tom."

After a verbatim transcript is prepared, information on nonverbal cues and other external factors not evident in the written transcript can be added and marked in the transcript using the assistant moderator's notes. Items to include are references to statements made with sarcasm or in jest, or a notation that "everyone was nodding their heads in agreement." Any relevant nonverbal and environmental factors that were noted may be added to assist in analyzing the discussion in its proper context.

Once the final transcript is prepared, the data can be analyzed using various approaches. Two common and relatively simple approaches used are *cut and paste* and *coding.* Using a cut and paste approach, which is more practical for smaller numbers of transcripts, the analyst reads the transcripts and marks the text for important ideas and quotes to be used. These sections of the text are then lifted from the text and placed together sequentially by topic area or grouped according to similar themes.[3] For example, when transcripts from a set of focus groups surrounding HIV prevention were analyzed, sections of text within each transcript which referenced reasons why people might engage in high risk behavior were cut from the transcripts and reassembled in a separate file. This allowed the analyst to see common themes and ideas relating to reasons why people might engage in high risk behavior across the series of focus groups. In addition, the discussions surrounding why people may take risks often led to discussions about how to reach risk-takers with prevention messages, which was another major topic area within the discussion. The analyst was able to cut select references to prevention messages for risk-takers in the "why people take risks" section, lift them from their original transcripts, and reassemble them along with text references in the "prevention messages" section. In the cut and paste method, quotes can be grouped separately for ease of reference when writing the final report.

In a coding approach, as the analyst identifies important ideas in the transcript, a label or code is attached to the specified portion of the text and placed in the margin of the transcript. Similar ideas receive the same, or closely, related codes.[2] For example, if a set of focus groups surrounding the topic of cardiovascular disease were conducted, a set of codes may emerge in reference to risks for cardiovascular disease. Sets of codes in this scenario might include codes related to nutrition and family history. Any textual references related to overeating, dietary fat, or foods high in fat or calories are examples of items which may receive a "nutrition" code. Similarly, references to family history of high blood pressure, high cholesterol, or heart disease may receive a "family history" code.

After the codes are assigned in a transcript, the analyst can review them and pull together all references to a single code or to any combination of codes.[2] In the sample cited above, the analyst may select all nutrition codes and specifically analyze those references in the transcript, or may combine the nutrition codes with any other codes in the text in order to suit the purpose of the analysis.

A variety of computer programs are available to assist in the analysis of qualitative data, including programs that will assist in managing and expediting the coding approach. Time and budget considerations, as well as access to computer programs, should be factored into the selected method of data analysis.

A third method of analysis, which can be less time-consuming, is to perform a tape-based analysis. In a tape-based analysis, the analyst reviews the discussion tapes and references the assistant moderator's notes to prepare a modified transcript.[2] This method is advantageous if time is limited and a brief, less-detailed final report is required.

TIPS AND TECHNIQUES FOR SUCCESS

There are several key steps that can easily be taken to ensure success when implementing a focus group project. These steps include (1) advanced distribution of the agenda, (2) incentives, (3) collecting demographic data, and (4) maintaining confidentiality.

Advanced Agenda Distribution

Prior to conducting a focus group, advanced distribution of the agenda, including main discussion topic areas and key questions to be asked by the moderator, may foster discussion and encourage all participants to share ideas. The agenda can be mailed with the confirmation letter or distributed a few minutes before the focus group discussion begins. If mailed with the confirmation letter, instructions should be included asking participants to identify points they may want to share during the discussion. Some participants will not complete the task, or may forget to bring the agenda along. As an option, the moderator may consider allowing five minutes before the focus group discussion begins to distribute the agenda and offer a few minutes for participants to quietly write down any ideas they may wish to share in the discussion.

Incentives

Although there are no guarantees that participants will attend, steps can be taken to decrease the number of no-shows. Offering incentives increases the chances that confirmed participants will come to the focus group. Cash incentives are commonly offered for focus group participation, but other alternatives, such as gift certificates, can also work. Gift certificates can be offered from a number of businesses such as beauty salons, hardware or sporting goods stores, restaurants, and movie theaters. For example, with a focus group consisting of mothers who will be exploring reasons why they chose not to breast-feed, or why they stopped breast-feeding soon after initiation, formula or coupons for formula, bottles, or other baby items might serve as effective incentives. Members of racial or ethnic groups should be consulted with regard to appropriate incentives for a particular population.

Some agencies may have policies which restrict or limit the types of incentives that can be offered to participants. This can often be addressed by writing a well-thought out proposal that references the importance of providing incentives to encourage and increase participant attendance. A detailed budget will reflect the cost of incentives in relation to the more costly expenses involved in conducting focus groups, such as moderator compensation, transcription, and data analysis.

Offering food to participants is another incentive for attendance. This is particularly important for focus groups that are held at night because participants may otherwise miss the evening meal. Food can be offered prior to the start of the focus group or after its completion. It is important not to interrupt the focus group to break for a meal because participants might talk about the topic during the meal, and some of the conversation may be missed if the taping equipment is turned off.

Assistance with child care may also increase attendance. When confirming participants, the recruiter determines if child care will be needed during the time the individual will participate in the focus group. In some cases, a licensed day-care provider may be willing to offer child care in another room at the site of the focus group. This possibility can be explored ahead of time and a price negotiated after estimating the number and age of children who will be requiring care.

In some cases, restrictions against offering child care could be encountered due to liability issues. Some participants may feel more comfortable leaving their children with their own day care provider or baby sitter than with someone they, and their children, do not know. In these situations, it may best to budget a reasonable amount for child care expenses to offer participants. This can be paid to the participant upon completion of the focus group, at the same time the incentive is given. A local child care licensing and training agency can help determine the average cost of care per child for a particular area. This will assist in determining a reasonable amount to offer participants who need assistance.

Demographic Data

After the focus group discussion has been completed, demographic data from the participants can be easily collected. A simple, one page form covering key demographics can be quickly completed by participants and easily compiled. A composite profile of participants involved in each focus group is beneficial during analysis and reporting. For example, if no participants with low household incomes or within a certain age range were involved in any focus group, this can be reported as a limitation in the generalizability of the results.

Confidentiality

Steps need to be taken to maintain participant confidentiality. No names, addresses, telephone numbers, or social security numbers should be placed on demographic sheets. Lists of participants need to be kept separate from any focus group transcripts and reports. Names of participants in groups should not be shared verbally or in writing. If the agency record-keeping policy allows, any records identifying participants and all focus group tapes should be destroyed as soon as the final report has been issued.

STRATEGIES FOR OVERCOMING BARRIERS

One of the most common barriers to implementing a focus group project is the considerable amount of time involved in administering each step in the process. One way to overcome time constraints is to contract out for services. If this option is pursued, the contractor needs to have a complete understanding of the entire project and expected outcomes. Time lines and budgets need to be developed and followed. The products that are expected from the contractor must be clearly outlined in detail. Communicating at regular intervals, and during implementation of key steps in the process, lessens the chance of error or oversight of critical elements by either party.

Another common barrier to focus group success is lack of transportation for participants. Public transportation vouchers or tokens can be provided if the focus group will be held within the public transportation system's hours of operation. If the focus group is held in an area with inadequate or limited public transportation, as is the case in many rural communities, alternatives such as a shuttle service, transportation by the sponsoring organization, or transportation by volunteers can be arranged. With the issue of transportation comes the issue of liability. By working closely with the sponsoring agency and with transportation providers, potential liability and how best to address the issues specific to the local circumstances can be determined.

EXPECTED OUTCOMES

Communicating the results of focus group research largely involves putting together the major findings of the study in a format easily comprehended by the intended audience. A written report detailing the project should incorporate many of the same elements included in the initial project proposal. Suggested elements to include in a written report are presented here, although a countless number of variations may be used depending on the scope of the project and the intended audience.

The report should include an introduction, methods, results, discussion, and recommendations. An introduction should identify the sponsor and coordinator of the project and the purpose of the focus group research. The introduction also describes the rationale for selecting the focus group technique as a means of data collection. If the results are to be used in conjunction with other forms of data collection, a brief description of the other methods, and how the data will be used together, should be provided.

The focus group method, including its strengths and limitations, needs to be presented in a separate section of the report. The methods section not only describes the focus group technique as a research method, but also includes information on the specific steps taken in the project. Information on data recruitment techniques, moderator selection, and logistics fit nicely into this section. Items for special consideration might also be presented here, or in another section. These items may include references to difficulties in data analysis, such as inadequate taping equipment that produced inaudible tapes. Other considerations that were made during analysis, such as recognizing that transcripts had been translated from a foreign language, should caution readers that some of the meaning or context may have been lost in translation. Any elements that may have potentially influenced the results, problems, or unexpected occurrences that were encountered and that are relevant to the outcome of the focus group results, and moderator observations can be presented here.

The section that presents the discussion results will be the lengthiest, most detailed segment as this is the heart of the report. An overall summary of results across focus groups may be given or broken down into results by focus group, topic area and question, or demographics if several demographic groups were studied. Any combination of the above may also be used. Determining the format depends on the type of information requested by the sponsoring agency, audience, nature of the topic and discussion, and writer's preference and style. There are no hard and fast rules about presenting results, leaving much room for flexibility and creativity. No matter which format is used, it is a good idea to use direct quotations, presented in their proper context, in the report. Nothing speaks louder than participants' own words.

A section on recommendations for action may be included in the report if the data analyst or writer was specifically asked to offer recommendations based on the data analysis. The focus group project sponsor may only want a report of the data and will take action on the findings when other elements are considered, such as findings from other qualitative or quantitative research.

CONCLUSION

The focus group method is quickly becoming a common practice in several health and human service agencies and in private and public organizations. Because focus groups allow for obtaining the qualitative viewpoints of target populations, many community-based coalitions are using focus group data for planning and evaluation. A thorough understanding of the focus group process will be beneficial to any health education or health planning practitioner. Numerous texts on focus groups and qualitative research are available for further reading, including the references used for this chapter.

References

1. Morgan, D. L. (1997). *Focus groups as qualitative research* (2nd ed.). Sage University Paper, Qualitative Research Methods Series, Vol. 16. Newbury Park, CA: Sage.

2. Krueger, R. A. (1994). *Focus groups: A practical guide for applied research* (2nd ed.). Thousand Oaks, CA: Sage.

3. Morse, J. M., & Field, P. A. (1995). *Qualitative research methods for health professionals* (2nd ed.). Thousand Oaks, CA: Sage.

Chapter 4

FACILITATING MEETINGS

Jean M. Prout, M.A., C.H.E.S.

Author's Comments: *Over the past 17 years, I have had the pleasure of working with many types of committees and experimenting with different types of facilitation. It has been extremely rewarding to start with an idea and utilize the expertise and assistance of a committee in order to produce a successful program. It is my sincere desire that this chapter will serve to provide you with concrete steps necessary for exemplary facilitation. Now more than ever, your leadership skills and diligence are necessary for committees to be efficient and productive. You will frequently be involved with a variety of committees and I hope you find that responsibility to be both challenging and rewarding. I encourage you to learn all you can about committees and their potential. Your position as a health educator empowers you to be an effective facilitator!*

INTRODUCTION

Health Educators are visibly involved with the complex activity of group dynamics. They take part in planning, facilitating, and evaluating a variety of group processes including meetings, conferences and workshops. One of their most important functions and most frequently used role is that of facilitator.

A common definition of facilitate is "to promote, aid, simplify, make easy." For a health educator, facilitation concentrates primarily on procedure and process, not on content. In some instances, too many facts might impede the decision making process of a group. On the other hand, too little information may also serve as a stumbling block. Therefore, it is important to be adequately familiar with the topic in order to facilitate the discussion.

This chapter provides guidelines for successful small group leadership. Included are descriptions of different types of committees and the steps necessary to obtain the type of group involvement that produces results. Committees will be highlighted as these are one type of small group that a health educator is likely to facilitate (e.g. community coalitions, department work-group committees).

TYPES OF COMMITTEES

As a facilitator, health educators participate in various community committees. They may guide an existing committee with members in place, or create a new committee that would most accurately accomplish designated goals. In general, health educators participate in the following types of committees: (1) Ad hoc committee, (2) committee-of-the-whole, (3) advisory committee, (4) task force, and (5) steering committee.

Ad Hoc Committee

An ad hoc committee is a temporary group that is established from within a larger committee. It has a specific purpose and a predefined deadline. For example, if a health educator were asked to design an innovative family planning clinic for an under-served rural population, an ad hoc committee could be assembled from members of the main family planning coalition to assist with the implementation of the clinic. After the ad hoc committee had made its recommendations, it would be recognized for the time and effort expended, and then disbanded.

The decision to create an ad hoc committee should be made jointly by (e.g.) health educators, medical directors, supervisors, superintendents, and any stake holder with a shared interest in the health issue at hand. Doing so will ensure that responsibilities are clear, implementation is smooth, and duplication of effort is alleviated.

Committee-of-the-Whole

The committee-of-the-whole is a discussion group that provides an opportunity for members of a board to ask questions pertaining to certain issues that may or may not be on the agenda. It is either held in conjunction with a regular board meeting (e.g., the Board of Directors for a local health department), or at a special meeting held for a specific purpose (e.g., determining if fees for family planning services should be increased). The committee-of-the-whole consists of interested board members who would like to discuss certain topics, without the formalities of the entire board. This type of meeting is not used for formal action or decision making, but simply to discuss issues pertaining to a decision. Health educators can serve as facilitators or resource persons for this type of committee.

Advisory Committee

At one time or another, nearly every health educator will have a need to solicit information from specific populations. An advisory committee, consisting of qualified members from the target population, serves as a mechanism for the health educator to obtain information by discussing issues that pertain to the target group. Members serve a specified term and are aware of the responsibilities of their commitment. An example of an advisory committee would be one that was created to discuss the implementation of a public act in a local school district (e.g., mandatory HIV education).

An advisory committee is one of the most powerful and effective committees a health educator can use for the group decision-making process. Not only does the advisory committee feel vitally important (due to their involvement with the project), their commitment leads to the desired ownership necessary for program success.

Active involvement by each person on the committee is necessary to achieve the facilitator's goals. It is important, however, for committee members to understand the advisory and temporary nature of their role from the beginning. Their position, however temporal in nature, will have long-lasting effects on the community.

Task Force

A task force is usually assembled by a facilitator for the purpose of completing a specific task. For example, a task force would be a viable committee to assist with a health fair at an elementary school, arrange for volunteers for a blood drive, or help publicize an upcoming event. The health educator serves as the facilitator to provide leadership and, in many cases, contributes the resources the group would need. The task force donates the human power, it does the "work." Once the defined goal or "task" is accomplished, the task force is discontinued. The facilitator should evaluate the task force's performance, as it may be reconvened at a later date for a similar commission.

Steering Committee

Steering committees oversee the process of implementing new programs. For instance, a steering committee could be used to assist in establishing protocols for soliciting, recruiting, and organizing volunteers. The steering committee consists of community members who have the skills necessary to perform the task. Each population group affected by the new program should have representation on the steering committee.

Members of the steering committee organize subcommittees to address various topics or programs. The number of subcommittees (also called ad hoc committees) is determined by the array of volunteers needed and the total sum of programs to be implemented. The facilitator organizes and works with the main steering committee which delegates assignments to subcommittees. Each subcommittee is disbanded once it has accomplished its specific purpose (e.g., a health program, such as a hypertension screening clinic, mammography screening program, stress management class, or a weight loss session).

ROLES OF THE FACILITATOR

Being involved with some aspects of the group process is an every day activity for health educators. Facilitation of the group process, however, can be difficult. What makes it so difficult is not the knowledge level of the health educator, but the need for flexibility and consistency in dealing with the impetuous nature of any committee. The health educator must learn to be a productive leader by developing the passion necessary to facilitate a committee as it works together to achieve a number of goals.

The manner by which the health educator facilitates, and the behavior that is modeled, will directly impact the interaction process of the committee. In his book, *Groups That Work (and Those That Don't)*, Richard Hackman, a well known scholar in the field of small group research, illustrated the importance of this modeling role. In trying to resolve the problems that a committee experienced due to his ineffective leadership ability, he concluded: "By finally modeling in my own behavior what I expected from others, I was able to rescue what many members were beginning to feel was a doomed project."[1] Exemplary facilitation therefore, demands an exemplary facilitator.

What distinguishes an effective facilitator from one who is not competent? Generally speaking, exemplary facilitators possess a non-judgmental, genuine and helpful attitude, and are able to (1) establish committee membership, (2) effectively plan meetings, (3) develop agendas, (4) publicize meetings, (5) keep committee discussion on task, (6) demonstrate appropriate conflict management skills, (7) attend to meeting formalities, and (8) keep a committee effective. Each will be described in further detail. In addition, many other excellent resources exist that can aid the reader in developing facilitation techniques.[2-5]

Facilitator Attitudes

For effective facilitation to take place, one element of extreme importance to health educators is their attitude. An attitude is a predisposition to behave in a certain way.[6] The way a facilitator responds to the committee, tasks, or a specific individual, directly impacts the group's effectiveness. So, what is the right attitude for a facilitator? In essence, there are several necessary attitudes for health educators to possess, including a genuineness in their interactions with others, a nonjudgmental attitude, a willingness to assist committee members, and an attitude of inquiry.

An Attitude of Genuineness

Integrity and authenticity are two of the most desirable traits a facilitator can possess. As facilitators, health educators need to display honesty when interacting with others. They should not rely on deception or coercion to obtain involvement, as members of the committee will quickly see through it. Insincerity is counterproductive, as individuals will either anticipate it or be irritated by it.[7] It is important to realize that power struggles and manipulation lead to a lack of confidence and low levels of trust between members of any group, which results in an inability to function.

An Attitude of Nonjudgment

Remaining neutral while facilitating a committee is easily said, but difficult to achieve. The facilitator must be open-minded with respect to the content of the discussion and needs to consider each idea on its own merit.[8,9] Health educators must avoid involvement with any slanderous small talk that easily develops within groups. The higher the amount of trust between committee members, the higher the capacity for learning and, thus, the greater the level of group effectiveness.[1]

With situations in which facilitators wish to contribute to group discussion, they should make it clear that they abandon the facilitator role for the moment in order to make a comment or present an idea.[10] The facilitator should present the information and then let the group decide if they want to discuss or disregard it.

An Attitude of Assistance

Effective facilitators desire to support and assist members in accomplishing their tasks. This is not to say that health educators "help" the group by solving their problems. Facilitators have to be extremely careful in "helping relationships" because self-reliance (i.e., the ability to act on one's own initiative), is important to each group member.[11] Appropriate facilitator support entails helping a committee member accept ownership of a problem and then correcting it with them. For example, if a news release was sent out too late to be effective, the facilitator should ensure that the committee member responsible for the delay realizes the problem and takes the necessary steps to rectify the situation.

An Attitude of Inquiry

Asking questions is an excellent communication technique the facilitator can use to enhance committee discussion. If information is requested by the facilitator when points are unclear, the committee will be able to avoid misunderstandings and a false feeling of agreement pertaining to decisions being made. When adequate deliberation is not allowed by the facilitator, the committee may pass a motion or have apprehensions about the pending decision. To ensure each member is understood, the facilitator should apply diversified communication skills (i.e., active listening, "I" messages). Keep in mind that any inquiry must be done from the right perspective (i.e., a position of curiosity, one of learning and of consideration). If communication is encouraged, a cooperative and effective decision will likely be reached by the committee.

Establishing Committee Membership

Facilitators need to recognize why an individual is either currently a committee member or willing to serve on a committee. There are personal motives involved with committee participation and several need to be considered prior to choosing new members. Does a recruit want to win approval, obtain prestige, gain knowledge, or develop skills? Is there a dedication to the committee's purpose? As an individual is considered for membership, facilitators must examine their expertise and abilities. Effective committee members have a variety of attributes including the following:

- They depend on the support and expertise of one another.

- They are a source of stimulation and communicate freely.

- They want to be included and are willing to commit the time and exertion necessary.

- There is a sincere allegiance for the committee's mission and goals; a desire for achievement.

When individuals have the aforementioned qualities, they are viable candidate for committee membership. To avoid misunderstandings with a potential member, a facilitator needs to clearly communicate four criteria: (1) The purpose of the committee, (2) type of committee, (3) duties of the membership, and (4) time commitment required. These specifications should be clarified when an individual is initially contacted and then clearly spelled out again in a letter of invitation.

The success or failure of a committee depends on the qualifications of its facilitator and his or her role in the selection of committee members. Health educators should incorporate a diversified membership strategy when recruiting members and take advantage of the opportunities to solicit support from local organizations (e.g., public or private associations, local schools, parent-teacher organizations, church groups, and special populations). Once the membership is in place, the facilitator is ready to plan a meeting.

Planning the Meeting

Planning a meeting is a complex activity. Five questions need to be considered to determine if a meeting is the most effective format for obtaining committee goals.

- What is the purpose of the meeting?
- Who should attend?
- Where should the meeting take place?
- When should the committee convene?
- How long will the committee continue?

There are times, however, when a committee meeting is not appropriate or possible. Examples of situations include, but are not limited to, the following:

- There is a need for immediate action and time does not allow for members' involvement.
- The committee decides the goal or mission is beyond their expertise.
- A goal or decision is not up for committee deliberation.
- Conflict management will need to take place and a meeting would be ineffective.

Developing the Agenda

Prior to each meeting, the facilitator needs to plan a meeting agenda. The printed agenda determines the content and the sequence of important events for the committee to discuss. It is imperative that the facilitator structure the agenda with "running clock" time allotments (e.g., 2:00 to 2:10 p.m.). Using time allotments, committee members will know what to expect and can easily follow whether or not the facilitator is adhering to the agenda. A lack of time assigned to agenda items may imply the necessity for a subsequent meeting.

The facilitator should ensure that agenda planning is done with committee members and any entity having an interest in the committee's activity. Less controversial or easier-to-handle and informational committee items should be placed early in the agenda, in order of increasing difficulty. Once easier decisions have been made, members feel more confident and can deal with more difficult issues. The business portion of the agenda (e.g., unfinished business, new business) should be structured with items requiring serious committee discussion placed in the middle of the agenda. This provides time for latecomers to arrive before important issues are discussed. After difficult items have been dealt with, the committee can move on to lighter items for discussion and generation of ideas. See Table 4-1 for a typical agenda format.

The agenda has three basic applications: (1) Ensure members are aware of new issues to be covered and have the time needed to research these items prior to the next meeting, (2) serve as a guide for the facilitator in leading the meeting, and (3) alert members to items that might need follow-up. When the agenda is received by members prior to the meeting, all three purposes will be accomplished. If the facilitator distributes the agenda to members at the start of the meeting, it is still of assistance, but effective participation by the members will be significantly reduced.

Committee members can modify an agenda, but this is not likely to occur if the agenda is carefully prepared and contains current items of business, as well as those decisions that need continued deliberation. Members have a vested interest in items on the agenda because of the time spent prior to the meeting preparing to discuss specific items. If the agenda is modified (e.g., items are deleted), committee member preparation is wasted, at least for that particular meeting.

Once the format for a group's agenda is determined, it is important to use the same outline for each subsequent meeting. The format should be general in nature so that all items requiring attention fall somewhere within the scope of the itinerary. This consistency serves a dual purpose: (1) Committee members and the public are assured that all meetings will follow a definite plan of order, and (2) the facilitator will have a predetermined outline to follow for each regular meeting. To more thoroughly understand the role of the agenda and how one is created, a copy of *Robert's Rule's of Order* should be obtained.[12] Descriptions for duties, procedures, motions, quorums, voting, nominations, and other necessary considerations are included. As these vary depending on committee type, they will not be discussed further here.

Table 4-1. Typical Agenda Format

I.	Call meeting to order
II.	Roll call of members
III.	Approval of minutes
IV.	Communications received
V.	Visitors present
VI.	Facilitator's report
VII.	Unfinished business
VIII.	New business
IX.	Adjournment

Publicizing Meetings

Publicity for committee meetings should be done by the facilitator well in advance of the actual meeting date. Agendas and all relevant materials should be received by the members at least one week prior to the meeting. If there is a significant amount of reading material or if pre-meeting tasks have been assigned, the facilitator needs to decide when materials need to be received by committee members.

Once the members have received an initial notification of the meeting, a second contact should be made within four days from the first announcement. This follow-up increases membership attendance and preparation. Facilitators can use a variety of techniques for contacting committee members, including phone calls, e-mail messages, post cards, or announcements in local newspapers.

The media should be notified of meeting times and dates if the facilitator thinks it would be beneficial for them to attend. Committee members, however, need to always be notified of the meeting prior to the media and prior to an announcement in the paper. If media coverage is desired, reporters can be informed of the meeting well in advance. A committee member should be assigned to meet with the press when they arrive. If the press arrives late, the member should leave the room to brief them in order to avoid disruption. Because the media can be utilized in many ways with committees, health educators need to be familiar with media advocacy skills (see Chapter 8, "Media Advocacy"), and utilize the expertise of local reporters when needed.

Keeping Committee Discussion on Task

The facilitator must fully concentrate on the committee's deliberation as most conversations have a normal tendency to wander in many directions.[4] Not only do facilitators need to pose questions, they are responsible for keeping the group focused in relation to the original topic. It is not a concern if the dialogue wanders off target every once in a while, but it is the facilitator's role to get the discussion centered again for the group. The more difficult the task, the more repetitions there will be in the committee's discussion.[13]

To help the committee stay focused on their agenda and the decision-making process, the facilitator should periodically summarize what has been said. The facilitator who loses track of the group's direction or conversation, should not try to cover up the confusion or become defensive. Instead, the facilitator could question the committee (e.g., "What are we saying?" or "Where do you think we are going with these facts?"). A break might be useful at that point so the facilitator could consult a colleague or the committee's recorder. A summary of the conversation is an effective way to focus the committee prior to continuing the meeting following the break.

Conflict Management

It is generally recognized that conflict is a major deterrent for decision-making committees. Some facilitators feel that ineffective communication is the major cause of conflict. Others feel that the cause may be a personality clash, an individual's annoying behavior, a goal or value discrepancy, a lack of cooperation, poor leadership, or differences in the way tasks are completed. Facilitators work tenaciously with committees consisting of individuals with varying and opposing personalities. It is the facilitator's vigilance with the group that determines the committee's effectiveness.

It is the facilitator's task to create favorable conditions that will positively affect the process and, hence, the outcome of the committee.[1] Avoiding *all* conflict in the decision-making conversation of the committee is not the facilitator's goal. When a moderate level of controversy is allowed, the committee makes better decisions in which more members seem to agree. The effects of "concurrence seeking" (i.e., members want to please each other in all situations), has repeatedly shown that committees arrive at lower quality decisions when compared to groups in which controversy and disagreement were properly facilitated.[14]

Facilitators differ in the way they attempt to handle conflicts. The facilitator who withdraws from disagreement demonstrates the need to surrender or conform and ineffectively remain neutral when there is a need to exhibit a leadership stance. This conformity may be the most incompetent leadership trait a facilitator can exercise, as it settles nothing for the group and allows hostility to escalate.

What is the optimal method for handling conflict? Facilitators need to possess the attitude that they are going to do something to address the situation, regardless of the consequences. Problems are best solved through a systematic procedure with the committee. At times, a facilitator will make a problem-solving decision based on intuition or experience. To gain an understanding of the problem causing the conflict, the facilitator should contemplate the following questions:

- Is the problem based on opinion or fact?
- What is the problem's origin?
- Is the problem critical?
- What will be accomplished by addressing the problem?
- What are the chances of a solution?
- Who is involved?

Attending to Meeting Formalities

The importance of the meeting setting should not be overlooked. An attractive, comfortable setting is one that is readily accessible and fun to attend. The setting should promote a positive atmosphere—one in which committee members feel relaxed and are inspired to be productive. Unfortunately, much of this is not attended to in committee meetings. For example, refreshments are not offered, which in many cases are one of the major rewards of everyday meetings.

Facilitators need to carefully plan or delegate the planning of physical room arrangements. Certain criteria used for selecting the appropriate meeting room are listed in Table 4-2. The facilitator has the responsibility for arriving early to ensure chairs and tables, technological equipment, refreshments, handouts, and name tags are appropriately situated. Seating arrangements are also very important and can affect communication between members. The facilitator needs to decide which type of seating formation to use. The room arrangement for the committee meeting will, to some extent, be dictated by the number of members. A number of different meeting room arrangements can be found in Figure 4-1.

Keeping Committees Effective

Committee members want to assist with the assessment, planning, implementation, and evaluation of health-related programs. A committee exchanging ideas and expertise will produce more effective decisions than any one person alone. A successful committee is a group of people who function together by working collectively. If members were asked what

Table 4-2. Meeting Room Considerations

- Number of committee members
- Writing surface for members
- Audiovisual needs
- Electricity
- Additional tables/carts for supplies
- Lighting options
- Noise level
- Temperature control
- Time allowance
- Availability
- Handicap accessibility
- Location

Figure 4-1. Meeting Room Arrangements

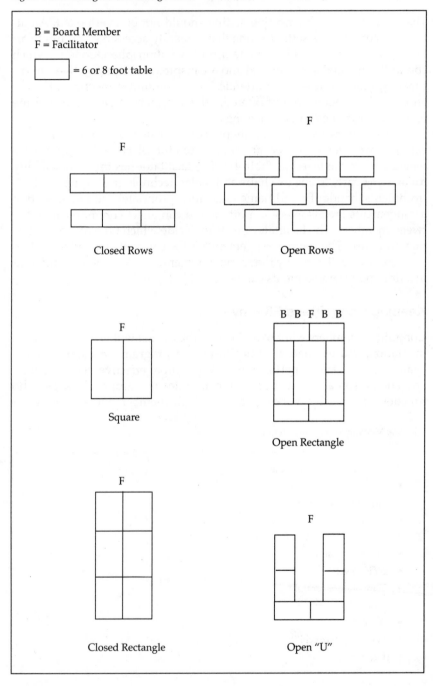

Figure 4-1 (continued).

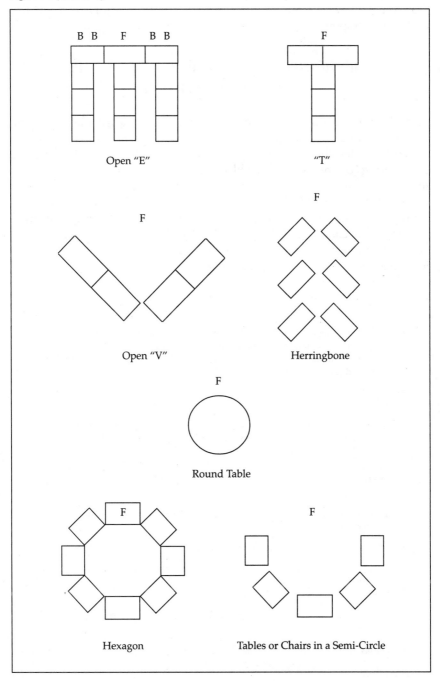

Open "E"

"T"

Open "V"

Herringbone

Round Table

Hexagon

Tables or Chairs in a Semi-Circle

they like about group involvement and committee meetings, the list in Table 4-3 would likely be identified. Facilitators should carefully read this list, and take each point into consideration as committees are planned.

DIFFERING COMMITTEE ROLES OF THE HEALTH EDUCATOR

As facilitators, health educators have an obligation to each committee member, their employer, and the community. When participating in various committee roles, the facilitator's responsibilities will change. In preparing for differing committee roles, health educators need to have an understanding of their own behavior. For instance, a health educator may facilitate one meeting, attend as a member, be a resource provider, and provide executive service. These changes in *position*, however, are rarely accompanied by actual changes in *behavior*. Even when health educators know what is expected of them in their various roles, they may not know the behaviors associated with these expectations.

Table 4-3. Characteristics of Effective Committees

- *Careful time management.* Time is a vital and carefully guarded commodity. Starting and ending on time is extremely important if the facilitator wants members to continue to attend meetings. Enough time should be allowed to finish the work and no more. Some facilitators designate a time keeper to help with this.

- *The facilitator and members are sensitive to each other's needs and expressions.* All members listen to and respect others' opinions.

- *Goals and objectives are clearly defined.* The committee's agenda, time frame, budget, planning, and evaluation procedures are understood by all members.

- *Interruptions at meetings are not allowed or are held to a minimum.*

- *The facilitator is prepared.* Materials are ready and available, both prior to and at the meeting.

- *There is a friendly, relaxed environment.* Even when the format is formal, there is an unassuming ambiance.

- *Members are qualified and have a vested interest in the committee's purpose.*

- *Accurate minutes or records are maintained.* Proper recording ensures decisions and results are accurate. Some facilitators designate a recorder to help with this.

- *Members feel validated.* Recognition and appreciation are given for various contributions.

- *The decisions or the propositions from the committee are actually used.*

Time needs to be allocated prior to each meeting to allow the health educator to plan for necessary role changes. A knowledge of the various roles a health educator assumes, and what the most effective types of communication are for each role will result in enhanced participation by the health educator.

CONCLUSION

Health educators have the fascinating opportunity to be the facilitators of various committees. At times they may ask if involvement is worth their time and effort. It may not seem like it during time-consuming decision-making, planning, implementation, and evaluation phases associated with diversified and numerous programs, but in the end, most find that committees positively impact program success. The satisfaction of seeing goals and objectives being achieved, and the positive results associated with facilitation is considerably rewarding. It makes all of the hard work, long hours, and unwavering dedication worthwhile.

References

1. Hackman, R. (1990). *Groups that work (and those that don't)*. San Francisco: Jossey-Bass.

2. Hart, L. (1992). *Faultless facilitation*. London: Kogan Page.

3. Heron, J. (1993). *Group facilitation: Theories and models for practice*. London: Kogan Page.

4. Jensen, A. & Chilberg, J. (1991). *Small group communication: Theory and application*. Belmont, CA: Wadsworth Publishing Company.

5. Phillips, L., & Phillips, M. (1993). Facilitated work groups: Theory and practice. *Journal of the Operational Research Society, 44*, 533-549.

6. Ajzen, I. (1991). The theory of planned behavior. *Organizational Behavior and Human Decision Processes, 50*, 179-211.

7. Gibb, J. (1960). Defensive communication. *The Journal of Communication, 10*, 141-148.

8. Broome, B., & Keever, D. (1989). Next generation group facilitation: Proposed principles. *Management Communication Quarterly, 3*, 107-127.

9. Keltner, J. (1989). Facilitation, catalyst for group problem solving. *Management Communication Quarterly, 3*, 8-32.

10. Doyle, M., & Straus, D. (1976). *How to make meetings work*. New York: Jove Books.

11. Schein, E. (1987). *Process consultation*. Reading, MA: Addison-Wesley.

12. Robert, H., III, & Evans, W. (1990). *Robert's rules of order*. New York: Harper Perennial.

13. Morris, C. (1966). Task effects on group interaction. *Journal of Personality and Social Psychology, 4*, 545-554.

14. Tjosvold, D. (1982). Effects of approach to controversy on superiors' incorporation of subordinates' information in decision making. *Journal of Applied Psychology, 67*, 189-193.

Chapter 5

COMMUNITY EMPOWERMENT

Leslie J. Bek, M.A.

Author's Comments: *It is my intent with this chapter to draw upon lessons I have learned in over 15 years of experience as a practicing health educator. In doing so, I am reminded of the time I first announced to my family that I was shifting my major to community health education. As I began to describe for them what exactly this meant in practical terms, I remember being somewhat unsure. I did know however, that I would be working with others to improve the health status of individuals and communities. And to me, that sounded both challenging and rewarding.*

My career has evolved from a hospital-based community health liaison, to health department staff educator, supervisor and administrator, to a university adjunct instructor, and finally to an independent consultant. Within my first six months as a staff health educator, I was involved in a new community health initiative. Our purpose was to bring together individuals, groups, agencies, and organizations with an interest in health promotion. Our Health Promotion Partnership would provide a monthly forum for increasing awareness, seeking assistance, and creating new activities and services that, as single entities, we could not have provided. Little did I know then that what we knew as collaboration, networking and cooperation, were really steps toward community empowerment.

Community empowerment is an initiative that has the potential to transcend disciplines and cultures. It brings together private, public, and nonprofit sectors of a community in a legitimate method for a commonly held purpose. Personally, I have encountered numerous rewarding relationships, experienced true partnerships, and developed a sense of kinship with empowerment team members. My professional vision has been broadened in a way that I would best describe as an awakening, whereas: "I'm the only difference between what is possible and what is impossible." In other words, an individual can become a conduit, a convener, or a catalyst in a community empowerment process, and the outcomes are limitless.

Empowerment is an enabling strategy analogous to the role of a coach. A coach enables the players or students by teaching fundamentals, outlining strategy, developing team work, building confidence, encouraging desire, and praising ambition. All positive steps toward a positive outcome. Empowerment can uplift with its potential. It can serenade like a symphony. Empowerment gives you confi-

*dence and energy like a sprinter, poised in the starting blocks, looking ahead, fo-
cused and ready. I view this chapter as my opportunity to coach you in community
empowerment strategy. And as your coach, I will take great pleasure in your future successes. Enjoy your journey.*

INTRODUCTION

Understanding the meaning of the term "empowerment" is important in
providing the framework for the understanding and application of community empowerment strategies. The essence of empowerment is "power."
For many, the concept of power is generally associated with strength, control, authority, and dominance over others. In contrast, the process of empowering others is "to give power or authority to . . . to give ability to . . . to
enable."[1]

Community empowerment is the process in which "individuals and
organizations apply their skills and resources in collective efforts to meet
their respective needs."[2] It provides a community with the capacity to set
priorities and control resources that are essential for increasing the
community's ability to determine its own persona. The sense of ownership
associated with this process makes communities more energetic, committed, and responsible.

Community empowerment includes two very basic actions: (1) Organizing a community in support of a common purpose, and (2) facilitating a process for integrating both traditional and nontypical systems and
networks in striving toward this purpose. Typically, empowerment is used
to shift public control to specific community entities, such as neighborhoods or residents in a housing district. Empowered communities have a
number of characteristics that differ tremendously from traditionally gov-
erned communities. In particular, empowered communities:[3]

- Are committed to their members.

- Understand and solve community problems.

- Are flexible and creative.

- Are effective in enforcing standards of behavior.

- Focus on capacities rather than deficiencies.

The context for health educators' involvement in community empowerment is defined in *Blueprint for a Healthy Community: A Guide to Local
Health Departments.*[4] This document introduced 10 essential elements to
protect and improve the health of communities; one of which is mobilizing
the community for action by providing leadership and initiating collabo-

ration. The capacity of a local health department to competently respond to this element involves empowerment. Strategies that embody skills and practices build capacity in practitioners and their community, resulting in community-driven mobilization.

A community empowerment strategy provides health educators, whose mission is to serve an entire community, with an opportunity to reach those whom they often seek to serve but so frequently miss. This is done by opening the doors and welcoming nontraditional members of the community into the discussions regarding planning, services and programs, to better address the community's needs. For example, if safety issues are a concern in a residential housing district, law enforcement officials and housing authorities should invite residents of the housing district and neighboring blocks to discussions regarding solutions. Making them equal partners in the process will help give insight into the problem, and provide a better solution. In essence, hierarchical levels of perceived power and authority are redefined to include nontraditional players. This strategy provides the opportunity for health educators to enhance the value and utilization of their agencys' services among community partners.

DEFINING THE COMMUNITY FOR EMPOWERMENT

The keyword, "community" provides challenges in terms of context. A community can represent people living in a geographic area, a subset of a larger group, or people in different locations sharing commonalities. The community itself, therefore, can be defined as many different environments. These environments can, for example, include a workplace, school district, church, county, city, or township. The communities with which health educators work are often defined by the jurisdictional boundaries of their employers (e.g., a county health department, a regional American Heart Association, a local school district, or company wellness plan).

To adequately provide services to meet the needs of individuals, health educators continually strive to identify individual target communities that exist within greater communities. In doing so, it is important to consider the community framework from the receiving end of services (i.e., the community's perspective) and consider the following questions: (1) Do the members of the defined community identify themselves as a community, (2) is the community a natural community (i.e., one in which people join for intrinsic reasons, such as a church or service club), and (3) would each member describe the relationship as one of community?

For example, a facilitator was hired to implement a community needs assessment process in two adjoining townships located in a rural, Midwestern county. The facilitator's employers saw these areas as readily established communities with township officials, town halls, and community centers. As efforts were initiated to create a team from within each township, a lesson was soon learned about the power of "practical and purposeful communities" (i.e., communities which evolve for a practical reason or purpose, such as a neighborhood watch effort, or an environmental action group). It was acceptable to think of each area in terms of township boundaries for issues such as taxing and zoning. When it came to assessing community needs, however, the perception of community was not consistent within established township boundaries. For some, the rural, three-mile dirt road on which they lived with their six neighbors defined their community. For others, community was defined by school boundaries. The only elementary school was located in Township A and was attended by both Township A and B students. After fifth grade, all students from both townships attended junior high and high school in Township B. Still others defined the community by who received the weekly newspaper, which was delivered only in a portion of Township B, and not at all in Township A.

Establishing a defined community in this case proved difficult. The facilitator quickly learned that the community needed to be defined from the community's perspective before empowerment strategies could be implemented. The focus of the community empowerment efforts began by finding "common unity" in establishing a community.

STEPS TO EMPOWERING COMMUNITIES

As with any health education process, effective community empowerment is a stepped procedure. Standard elements of any community empowerment include (1) creating the community empowerment team; (2) establishing a shared vision; (3) assessing needs, assets, and resources; (4) determining leadership roles; (5) building capacity; and (6) sustaining community relationships.

The following example will be used as an illustration of how these elements can be applied.

> Access to dental care for low income children was identified as a need in a rural county of 70,000 people with four population centers; the largest being 25,000 people. Continuing low rates of Medicaid reimbursement had forced local dentists to serve only existing patients and no longer accept new Medicaid patients. It was estimated that 6,000 Medicaid-eligible children were not receiving dental care due to this policy. It would take considerable effort to enact policy changes that would alleviate the access problems to dental care. Thus, the problem continued to mount as a no-win situation.

> *When a single parent of three children moved into the community and discovered there would be no dental coverage for her children, she initiated the community empowerment process. Three years later, the community opened the doors to the region's first public health dental clinic. The purpose of the clinic was to provide dental services to low-income and Medicaid eligible children.*

Creating the Community Empowerment Team

The community empowerment process should not be a solo effort taken on by a motivated health educator alone; it should be a collaborative effort consisting of interested and supportive community members. In the dental clinic example, the team consisted of representatives from the Dental Society, social services, Medicaid, the local health department, Head Start, a philanthropic foundation, and, most importantly, concerned parent advocates.

In choosing team members, the health educator should look for individuals who will contribute to the solution. Individuals with authority and policy makers are obvious first choices, as they possess clout in the community. Other community members with an interest in the empowerment process should also be invited to join. This can be done through personal letters, telephone calls, newsletters, or newspaper articles. It is important for the health educator to realize that potential members have varied amounts of time to commit to the empowerment effort. If members cannot attend meetings, they can still be oriented to the purpose or focus of the empowerment effort and assist indirectly with advocacy activities. Even team members involved at a minimal level must have an understanding of the issue.

Individuals, such as youth, older adults, people with disabilities, artists, and welfare recipients, are less likely to be considered when establishing an empowerment team, but can provide insight that would normally be overlooked. These individuals are often those targeted to receive community-based services, yet are never asked for their input. Local *associations* (e.g., neighborhood groups, religious institutions, cultural organizations) and local *institutions* (e.g., schools, police departments, hospitals, community colleges, parks, and libraries) should also be considered for the empowerment team. It is the blending of individuals, associations, and institutions that brings balance and strength to the empowerment process. While an *individual* becomes the member of the team, they actually can be a representative of a far greater partner. For example, a rural Midwestern empowerment team had a common goal of increasing access to medical care for uninsured and underinsured persons through the establishment of a new referral model. The Regional Medical Center (RMC) was represented on the team by an individual administrator. The primary challenge to the administrator, if she was to best *represent* her hospital, was to think globally in regard to the entire assets and resources of the RMC as they relate to the empowerment goal. Secondly, she would be called upon to communicate this message and advocate for support from the RMC to the extent to which she has committed them. The organizational support can also provide necessary credibility and clout to the process.

An empowerment team is sure to face a variety of challenges and should plan for them in advance. For instance, not everyone on the team will be supportive of all decisions. It is important that the concerns of those who oppose a decision are addressed. Differences may simply have been misunderstandings and, once resolved, opponents may end up joining the cause. While dealing with controversy, the process should not be allowed to become chaotic. It may be the strategy of adversaries to engage the community empowerment team in challenging "no-win" discussions. With these situations, time and energy are wasted, as the team has been deterred from its original goal of action.

This lesson was learned by a rural community during its focus on adolescent health issues. The team, led by the local health department, set out to assess current adolescent health status and needs. The process involved administering a health status survey, which had been developed by a local physician, to high school students. Some members of the community were convinced that the intent of the project was to establish school-based health clinics where condoms would be dispensed without parental consent. They believed the process was a smoke-screen and that a hidden agenda existed. This belief was fueled somewhat by the knowledge that the state government was funding school-based clinics in other regions of the state. Other local physicians feared that school-based clinics would divert patients from their practices. Opponents attended coalition meetings and exalted these opinions.

In this situation, it took additional time, energy, and patience to address the diversion attempt by the nay-sayers. It also took personal resolve by the team to remain "cool" when, for all appearances, some community members were essentially saying they did not believe the stated intent of the process or its results. A resolution was reached by developing a consensus document that stated the mission of the initiative and included clearly defined goals and objectives.

Other community members also can be instrumental to the community empowerment process, even if they are not directly involved with the empowerment team. This was found to be true with the dental care issue. For instance, a local United Way Director was invited to attend an informational meeting by the dental clinic's core development team, regarding the services provided by the clinic and its need for financial support from the community. The United Way itself could not provide financial assistance at that time, and it soon became apparent that it was unlikely the dental clinic would apply to become a member agency. Likewise, the United Way Director could not serve in an official capacity on the community empowerment team. The Director, however, had become a knowledgeable advocate for community issues. Several weeks later, when contacted by the local television news team for a lead on a youth health issue, the United Way Director immediately referred the reporter to the dental clinic. The result was an opportunity for the dental clinic to share its story directly to its constituents on an evening news program.

Establishing a Shared Vision

In many aspects, the empowerment process, mirrors the health education program planning process. A defining element in empowerment is the role of the target community in creating and sharing a vision. It is critical that the purpose for which the community is rallying originates from within, and is accepted by the community.

Effective team leaders begin by establishing, with the empowerment team, a vision, or goal for the future. This vision is the hallmark of effective empowerment team building. It makes the process worthwhile, and ensures team members will be eager to participate.

The empowerment goal must be shared by all community empowerment team members. In a survey of 75 empowerment teams, it was found, without exception, that the teams that were functioning effectively had a clear understanding of their objectives.[5] Successful empowerment teams also had ownership of the goal to be achieved and a belief that the goal embodies a worthwhile and important result in the community. Conversely, a team's ineffectiveness in the empowerment process usually stemmed from (1) an unfocused or politicized goal, (2) a lost sense of urgency, or (3) personal goals superseding team goals.[5]

The organizers of the dental care issue believed that dental care was a community need and promoted the message that the situation needed a community solution. In the process, team members did not want to alienate dentists and make them out to be part of the problem. In fact, many dentists in the area had been providing a community service by subsidizing the care of low income children and Medicaid eligible patients. The result was a "win-win" situation for the following reasons: (1) The vision was compatible with the dentists' professional ethic of assuring that dental services were accessible to all children in need; (2) the dentists did not have to continue to endure financial losses; and (3) the dentists continued to provide services to their current low income patients, while eventually voluntarily serving as advisory board members to the new dental clinic. Further, some dentists lent support by serving and actively soliciting contributions to the dental clinic as empowerment team members.

The importance of the shared vision can not be overstated as it serves as the rallying cause at the start of the process and shall be the centering point to which the team shall return throughout the process. Determining the shared vision is a task of the empowerment process during its infancy. And like other experiences in developmental stages, the process of reaching agreement can have lifelong implications. The following steps demonstrate one method for establishing a shared vision:

1. Before beginning a discussion of the issue, teams of two can interview each other, taking turns as questioner and responder to the following two questions: (1) What motivates you to be involved in this process? and (2) what do you want to accomplish the most through your involvement?

2. After the interviews, time should be allowed for introducing each other and identifying what was learned about their partners' motivation and expectations for accomplishment.

3. While listening to the reports of these interviews, the words and phrases that appear to be most significant should be noted.

4. Using these words and phrases, sentences can be written that begin to reflect the group's vision.

5. The resulting piece is a vision in first draft form that can be the basis for further discussion and refinement by the team.

Assessing Needs, Assets, and Resources

The process of assessment brings order to the community empowerment process. An assessment process establishes a baseline, sets parameters, and begins to define tangible frameworks within the community. In addition, it provides a system of analysis that allows for close scrutiny of the community components. Throughout the assessment, the team's vision of the issue broadens. Potential new team members or supporters are identified through the process of determining assets and resources. Assessment reassures members that the community empowerment process has a logical pathway for accomplishing its goals.

During the assessment process, emphasis should be placed on assessing assets and resources. *Assets* are strengths of a community, such as wide support for safe and drug free schools, low teen pregnancy rates, low school dropout rates, strong family support and involvement, and low crime rates. *Resources* are more traditional and tangible, such as financial support, or structural facilities in the community. Traditional processes tend to determine community needs from a problem-focused base. These processes implement a crisis-management style that concentrates on reducing or alleviating problems. What is needed is a shift in thinking to asset building. Asset-based assessment is positive and leads to creative solutions that utilize available resources. Traditional problem-based thinking emphasizes needs that often require additional, scarce financial resources.

Social research results focusing on community empowerment strategies to benefit youth have shown the value and potential of building assets within the community. In one case, 30 developmental assets, including family support, social competencies, and discipline were identified as essential elements for a healthy community comprised of healthy youth.[6] Just like ensuring that the target population has a community identity, assets, rather than perceived problems, should be determined. Assets will not only reduce the scope of the empowerment challenge, they will become part of the solution. This is because, like dollars (a financial asset), strengths, such as word processing skills, can become a part of the solution, reducing the dependence on new dollars.

The popularity of an asset-focus model should not fully overshadow the traditional identification and utilization of resources. Because strengths build on and use available resources, it is essential to have an awareness of the resources that exist within the community. A nice problem to have would be community empowerment team members debating whether something is an asset or resource.

Determining the Leadership Role: Institutional Versus Situational

In the community empowerment process, there can be both institutional leaders and situational leaders. Initiatives that generate community empowerment often involve *institutional leaders* (e.g., County Commissioner, agency director) by necessity. These individuals give the effort clout and a sense of priority to the community. Because institutional leaders are in positions of responsibility for some aspect of community welfare, they often hold resources that can fuel the project. Additionally, they hold the decision-making authority to create change. Company or agency CEOs are great institutional leaders, because they are usually skilled analysts and knowledgeable about policy formation and interpretation. They are accustomed to a hierarchical system, running an organization, and establishing a budget. However, not all potential institutional leaders are right for the position. The following questions concerning their abilities should be assessed by the empowerment team: (1) How does their institutional leadership role translate to a new situation outside of their comfort zone? (2) how successful are they as team players, versus as leaders? and (3) how do they function with a consensus decision-making model? Determining strengths and weaknesses prior to filling leadership roles is important. Once in the role, the situation can be sensitive and politically-charged. Ineffective leaders, in the role only because of their organizational positions, can suffocate an empowerment process.

Leadership roles may also involve *situational leaders*. These leaders usually hold staff positions within local organizations. In the community empowerment process, they act as coalition coordinators. Staff acting as situational leaders may sometimes find these positions outside of their comfort zones, as they may be challenged with directing and leading a process involving a group of institutional leaders. Due to both their training and expertise, health educators are excellent candidates for serving as situational leaders.

Ideally, effective leaders possess the principles inherent in the Servant Leadership Model.[7] This model places service to others—including employees, customers, and community—as the number one priority. Besides emphasizing increased service to others, the Servant Leadership Model stresses a holistic approach to work, promotes a sense of community, and shares power associated with decision making. Characteristics of servant leaders are listed in Table 5-1.

It is important to remember that the leader will also be challenged to stay abreast of the team members' thoughts and feelings. Expectations of individuals will be different, and tolerance levels will vary. If the team mood

Table 5-1. Characteristics of Servant Leaders

- *Listener*. Will listen to the group and reflect on their thoughts.

- *Empathetic*. Strive to understand and empathize with others as people need to feel valued and rewarded.

- *Healer*. Possess a healing influence on oneself and others.

- *Aware*. Have an understanding of ethics, values, and a holistic point-of-view.

- *Persuasive*. Reach consensus via persuasion rather than coercion.

- *Conceptualizer*. Big vision, dreamer, think beyond the day-to-day.

- *Foresight*. Understand lessons from the past, realities of the present, and likely consequences of a decision for the future.

- *Stewardship*. Has the trust of others and of the greater community.

- *Belief in the growth of people*. People have intrinsic value that should be nurtured.

- *Belief in building community*. Recognize that abilities come from within organizations and institutions.

is not monitored, partners may be lost, damage control may be needed, and future partners may back out of the process. The leader should always remember the community empowerment process cannot be controlled; it can only be facilitated, inspired, and embraced.

Building Capacity

If a baseball team was being established, it would be assumed that recruits could at least throw and catch the ball. A need for capacity building means simply that some of the empowerment players brought their gloves, yet they cannot seem to stop a ground ball. What would seem to be for-sure outs are becoming base hits. In essence, the team is hurting itself. By working on basic skills related to fielding a ground ball, the team is more likely to make the plays in the future and, therefore, be more likely to achieve their team goals.

What expectations should be placed on community empowerment players? The community empowerment leader should expect new recruits to possess certain fundamentals, and build on these through extensive team training. These fundamentals would include a shared vision or common goal, a positive outlook toward goal attainment, flexibility and willingness to compromise, and knowledge of community assets and resources.

Residents of a community must have confidence in the empowerment team's ability to create the conditions in which they can meet empowerment goals. Health educators must possess skills that can assist residents in building confidence in both themselves and in the team's ability to provide direction to the process.[4] Building capacity, therefore, is a focus on training and is the lasting contribution that the empowerment process makes in the community. Capacity building skills that the health educator and team members need to possess include the following:

- *Decision making.* Methods of reaching consensus.

- *Record keeping.* Most important for documenting responsibilities for tasks, status, and outcomes.

- *Packaging the story.* To assure the same message is being communicated throughout the community and to facilitate effective communication, tools can be developed such as fact sheets, action plan grids, and mission statements.

- *Data analysis.* Specific skills are necessary to properly interpret health status rates, economic impact, or census data and contributing factors. Additionally, skills are needed in assessing data using increasingly advanced electronic and telecommunications mediums.

- *Sustaining the process.* Thought needs to be given to ongoing roles, responsibilities, and agreement reached on a team structure. Assurances must be made that the persons involved are "willing partners" and were not randomly assigned by others.

- *Communication.* An element of paramount importance when considering the mix of community empowerment team members, their backgrounds, and levels of comfort in voicing their opinions to the team.

- *Fund-raising.* An essential element that may make a significant contribution to the success of the impending community empowerment goal. Fund-raising is a task to which team members usually respond, "I will do anything other than ask people for money." Fund-raising skills must include the ability to determine target markets for fund-raising efforts, create a core development team, write fund-raising objectives, and train volunteers.

- *Assessment.* Determining assets and resources in a systematic way. Several models of assessment can be used.

- *Effective meeting management.* This capacity will provide immediate impact on the credibility of the empowerment process. If meetings are efficiently and effectively managed, they have a greater likelihood to positively affect individual participation.

- *Conflict resolution.* Many preventive tasks, such as predetermining decision-making procedures, and documentation of responsibility, will deter conflict. Skills will be needed, however, to respond to a myriad of "what if" situations.

A comprehensive primer of such capacity building processes and techniques is *Young People Creating Community Change.*[8] This how-to guide covers topics such as working in groups, managing time, generating program ideas, and creating an action plan.

Assets and resources may already exist in the community that can assist in training team members on capacity building. For example, an intermediate school district may provide training on small group facilitation, while local universities can assist with conflict resolution. All teams need practice to enhance their performance. Attention to capacity building assures fundamental bases of the empowerment team are covered.

Sustaining Community Relationships

The success of the community empowerment process depends on the development of structured relationships with empowerment partners. For many partners, an empowerment process is the first time they have talked or worked with others in the community. Participants will soon see the value of other team members' services and activities, which enhances the team's value and unity. All team members are challenged to sustain these relationships and to share positive empowerment experiences with the broader community. Sustaining relationships takes a commitment similar to that of nurturing a friendship. Plans need to be made to keep in touch or to reconvene as a group. This can be accomplished via various routes, such as creation of an advisory board, or quarterly or biannual update luncheons.

The dental clinic empowerment team was sensitive to sustaining relationships after services were a reality. A voluntary advisory board was created to provide governance and a continual community voice. The board consisted of three local dentists, a school district health coordinator, social services and Head Start representatives, and parents of clinic patients.

TIPS AND TECHNIQUES FOR SUCCESS

> *Good judgment comes from experience, and experience, well, that comes from poor judgment.* - Anonymous

The community empowerment process can be enhanced in a number of ways. In particular, establishing credibility and beginning with nonthreatening community issues will increase the likelihood that community empowerment goals will be achieved.

Establishing Credibility

It has been suggested that "it takes at least 20 rights to undo a single wrong." Damage control can be kept to a minimum by establishing credibility as a community empowerment team early in the process. Positive personal relationships between the team and the community will enhance the likelihood of community acceptance and trust. In addition, the community empowerment team must complete what it sets out to accomplish. Throughout the process, they must also give to and receive feedback from the community-at-large or special interest groups. Finally, the team must be accountable to the community. Accountability means being able to clearly state the vision, goals, and objectives of the empowerment process, and to rationalize actions taken to the community.

The involvement of the local dental society in the dental clinic example greatly enhanced the empowerment team's credibility within the community. The message was being sent that dentists, who had been providing under-compensated care to local children, were willing to invest time into finding a long-term solution. Because the community believed the dentists should be consulted and involved as partners, the team was seen as one that could expertly lead the process toward accessible dental services for all community children.

Beginning With Non-Threatening Issues

Even when a community empowerment initiative gains support and momentum, it can be risky. The tasks of creating a team and establishing a shared vision will be hastened if the team begins with nonthreatening issues. The team must consider that the community empowerment solution will ultimately require change. This has a potentially threatening impact on public and private sector community members who may be key players in the process. It is important to tread safely in the beginning as relationships and trust are developing. Areas of improvement about an issue that could be considered "small-wins" should be publicized. As the community gels and becomes part of the empowerment process, more controversial, time-consuming issues can be tackled.

From the beginning, the dental care empowerment process avoided finger-pointing and assigning responsibility for the dental services problem. The vision focused on empowerment, community assets, and healthy children, which kept key people involved with, rather than opposed to, the process.

STRATEGIES FOR OVERCOMING BARRIERS

Barriers to the community empowerment process should be preventable, or at the very least, "treatable." Typical barriers usually include (1) a lack of consensus among team members, (2) inadequate levels of awareness among team members as to the pertinent factors in goal attainment, and (3) a hampering of empowerment team members functioning at full capacity due to misinformation or misinterpretation. These barriers can be lessened by (1) developing communication skills, (2) setting realistic time lines, and (3) being flexible.

Developing Communication Skills

Development of effective communication skills is, by far, the most important strategy for preventing or overcoming potential barriers. The act of communication has also been referred to as the "art of communication." It is integral to the learning of empowerment skills, to the implementation of empowerment processes, and understanding of both team and community roles.

In order to gain community support, a story must be communicated. During the process, the team must continuously interact and communicate with the community. Elements of effective communication skills include the following:

- *Identifying channels of communication.* It is important not to reinvent the wheel. Being in tune with and utilizing existing channels of communication can be an asset to the empowerment process. Examples of existing communication channels may include electronic mail, television cable event calendars, newsletters, meeting minutes, GANTT charts, staff meetings, interagency meetings, and church bulletins.

- *Listening skills.* Especially in the team building process, care needs to be taken to listen, rather than just waiting for an opportunity to speak. Effective listening includes asking the person speaking to summarize what was heard and requesting confirmation of the message received.

- *Giving and receiving feedback.* Listening skills continue in what has been described as the "feedback loop." First, one must listen effectively in order to provide appropriate and constructive feedback. Secondly, one must listen effectively to the feedback that is given.

- *Written communication.* An awareness and understanding of the intended audience is always at the core of any method of communication. Implementation of a readability index will help in gauging the reading level of the written piece. Context and jargon should also be analyzed for community understanding.

- *Verbal communication.* Time must be taken to evaluate verbal communication outcomes. Body language, such as eye contact, smiling, and nodding, facilitate successful verbal communication.

- *Interpersonal skills.* A level of comfort between participants will go a long way toward enhancing all facets of communication. It will also enrich the trust factor of the working relationship.

Setting Realistic Time Lines

For most members, the empowerment effort will require additional time beyond jobs, family, and other obligations. Therefore, efficient utilization of time is important. Unrealistic time lines can have consequences on the overall process and will affect team credibility in the community. Community empowerment leaders should assume at the beginning of the process that procedures will take longer than expected, and plan accordingly. The rule is to adhere to a time line, and adjust it if necessary.

Being Flexible

The community empowerment process must be flexible. This flexibility can be illustrated as a willingness to modify time lines to accommodate new information or the training needs of team members. Flexibility also ensures all partners will be allowed to make individual contributions to the process and that their input can alter or modify its direction. The empowerment process can have definition, goals and objectives, but should remain flexible. There is no single, correct way to implement the empowerment process—it is totally dependent on the needs of the community and the empowerment team.

Evaluating the Empowerment Process

The concept of evaluation seems to invoke stress and tension in the real world. It carries the connotation of pass or fail that most people gladly left behind with their formal education. Mentioning the word evaluation to a community empowerment team may invoke many emotions from fear to excitement. Evaluation is, however, essential for determining the effectiveness and efficiency of empowerment efforts. An appropriate evaluation plan needs to be developed prior to the onset of the empowerment process. Because of the benefits associated with evaluation, it should be embraced rather than feared.

A first step is to simplify the mental model of evaluation for team members. The team already has the basic skills or knowledge for a level of evaluation that is practical. The leader should continue to simplify the process as the team begins to formulate an evaluation design. The following questions will guide the empowerment evaluation: (1) What does the team want to know? and (2) did the team do what they said they would? Process objectives, short-term impact, long-term outcomes and attitude, knowledge and behavior measures, can all be components of the community empowerment evaluation plan. Resources should be sought out, if necessary, to assist in finding an evaluation format that fits the team.

Evaluation results will have lasting benefits in the community and to those involved in the process, and is essential for building credibility and sustaining empowerment efforts. Reporting negative results should not be avoided, as reporting only the positive outcomes is cheating the community. The purpose of evaluation is not just to show what has been effective, but rather to help all involved learn from the community empowerment process, and to improve upon it for future empowerment endeavors.

EXPECTED OUTCOMES

Community empowerment should have defined expectations for what will be found at the end of the process. Goals and objectives should be set in order to measure later success. These should be measured both during implementation of the community empowerment process and after the process has been completed.

Hopefully, a positive community empowerment experience will stay with participants and be replayed in different settings, leading to positive results in the future. The long-term empowerment goal is to have sustained impact on changing community norms. An investment has been made by both the community empowerment team and the community. All team members need to be encouraged to use their experience to continue to guide community members toward change.

Sustaining the empowerment effort will also require a commitment by team members to future empowerment endeavors, such as following-up on the original actions, reassessing assets, resources and needs when necessary, and revising activities accordingly. Once it has been initiated, the community empowerment process is cyclical in nature; it truly has no end.

CONCLUSION

Community empowerment can be a challenging and powerful process. It has been common practice for "leaders" in communities to structure processes to solve problems by inviting themselves to meet on issues. These leaders are often the institutional leaders of the community. The result has been the development of a plan to solve other people's problems. The empowerment process, however, draws the "community experts" into the discussion and development of a shared vision.

The health educator assists in the community empowerment process by facilitating meetings and discussions, and helping to organize and plan activities chosen by the team. The community empowerment process is a call to action for the health educator, for if present systems were operating correctly, communities would be healthier than they currently are.

Depending on the issue to be addressed in the community empowerment process, sustainable change may take a period of time. Those involved in the process should expect a lengthy, but rewarding process.

References

1. Guralnik, D. B. (1974). *Webster's new world dictionary of the American language, second college edition.* Cleveland: William Collins, World Publishing Co.

2. Israel, B. A., Checkoway, B., Schulz, A., & Zimmerman, M. (1994). Health education and community empowerment: Conceptualizing and measuring perceptions of individual, organizational, and community control. *Health Education Quarterly, 21,* 149-170.

3. Osborne, D., & Gaebler, P. (1997). Reinventing government. In D. Osborne and P. Plastrik (Eds.), *Banishing bureaucracy: Five strategies for reinventing government.* Reading, MA: Addison-Wesley Publishing Co.

4. National Association of County Health Officials, & Centers for Disease Control and Prevention. (1994). *Blueprint for a healthy community: A guide for local health departments.* Atlanta: Centers for Disease Control and Prevention.

5. Larson, C. E., & LaFasto, F. (1989). *Teamwork: What must go right, what can go wrong.* Newbury Park, NJ: Sage Publications.

6. Benson, P. L. (1990). *The troubled journey: A portrait of 6th-12th grade youth.* Minneapolis: Search Institute.

7. Greenleaf, R. K. (1991). *Servant Leadership: A journey into the nature of legitimate power and greatness.* New York: Paulist Press.

8. Checkoway, B. (1996). *Young people creating community change.* Battle Creek, MI: W. K. Kellogg Foundation.

Chapter 6

PRESENTATION SKILLS

Heather M. Stys, B.S.

Author's Comments: *I often ask myself whether a good public speaker is born or made. Based on my experiences, I feel that it is a little of both. Some people naturally take to the art of performing. Getting up in front of a crowd of 250 people excites and challenges them. My concern, however, is for those individuals who have the potential to become dynamic speakers, but convince themselves that they just cannot do it. They become so intimidated with the performances of "natural" speakers that they lose the determination and drive to improve. I believe efforts should be made, particularly in the field of health education, to require a greater amount of public speaking experiences before entering the profession. The only way to "make" good speakers is to expose and re-expose them to a variety of situations. This allows them the chance to learn, correct, and solidify high quality speaking skills. Avoidance of this valuable lesson will surely be a detriment to our profession.*

INTRODUCTION

Proficient presentation skills are indispensable to a health educator. Public speaking provides an opportunity to impress, persuade, and sell others on concepts and ideas that directly impact individual and community health status. Public speaking should be a challenging but enjoyable process that, when properly planned for, can provide tremendous intrinsic and extrinsic rewards. Unfortunately, many health educators approach public speaking with trepidation. They view it as an obstacle that creates anxiety and stress. A health educator who dislikes public speaking makes about as much sense as a lactose intolerant person being an ice cream tester. Because a great deal of health education involves presenting information to target populations, it is essential that a health educator possess effective presentation skills. Having these skills not only alleviates anxiety, they increase the likelihood that the appropriate message is received by the audience.

Being truly effective with public speaking is dependent on a number of factors, including the effort that goes into the preparation of a presentation and the presenter's speaking skills. As with any health education process, preparing for a presentation can be time consuming and a difficult task. Should the blue suit be worn, or no suit at all? Will the audience find the experience exhilarating, or will they fall asleep? Should creativity be risked, or is simplicity the best bet? Although there are no definitive answers to these questions, effective planning and delivery skills can make the experience positive for both the presenter and the audience. It will involve some homework and hard work, but the final results are worth the effort. Through careful planning and preparation, a health educator can be effective in any speaking situation.

PREPARING FOR A PRESENTATION

Being aware of the surroundings and expectations of the audience is important in preparing for a presentation. This entails knowing the audience, topic, and presentation expectations. For instance, an audience could consist of young people in school, individuals attending a personal behavior change seminar, professionals attending a workshop, members of a community coalition committee, or community volunteers working as an advocacy group. Each group has needs and expectations unique to their situation. In order to elicit a desired response from listeners, information about them is needed, such as ages, occupations, religions, attitudes, beliefs, moods, and feelings.[1]

Health education topics could be centered around a specific topic, such as breast cancer, or focused on many areas, like general women's health. Presentation expectations are directly influenced by the setting in which the program takes place such as a boardroom, auditorium, classroom, or community center. Prior to the presentation, the health educator should find out who will be attending, what needs to be covered, and the time frame allotted for the presentation. A competent speaker should be ready for a variety of questions. Therefore, it is important that the speaker has thoroughly researched the need, developed objectives, and maintained open lines of communication with the coordinator of the presentation.

The following experience illustrates what can happen when a presentation has been poorly planned:

> I was asked to give a two-hour program for 20 females on women's health issues at a local correctional facility. The information came easily because of the programming I had done over the course of my career. My files had plenty of overheads, videotapes, and handouts. I never gave much thought to the target audience, what information would be best, how it would be best presented, and what the expectations of the instructor were. When I got dressed for work that morning, I put on my usual skirt, blouse, and blazer. As I arrived at the prison, it occurred to me that I was overdressed. The instructor even

commented on how "fancy" I appeared and asked if it would be all right if I would enter the classroom without the blazer. Embarrassed, I apologized. After entering the room, I gathered my handouts and began to pass them out. As it turned out, two women could not read and one spoke Spanish. The information was too complex and my appearance made it difficult for the participants to feel comfortable. If I had just taken the time to call and ask the instructor some basic questions, I would have saved myself some uneasiness and been able to center the program more around audience needs. It became a valuable lesson that I have carried from that point forward. Instead of addressing the issues beforehand of what to wear, which materials to bring, or if there were any special learning styles, I jumped in head first and ended up drowning.

Good speakers should also be able to adapt to their surroundings. Adaptation is necessary throughout the entire speaking process. For instance, the approach a health educator uses in talking about blood borne pathogens in a factory setting will be quite different than presenting to public health nurses at a health department. Speakers are able to better adapt when they consider audience composition, knowledge levels, and attitudes.[2] Speakers who get into the habit of gathering information prior to a presentation make better connections and impressions with their audiences and are more likely to adapt to meet the needs of the audience.

Understanding Different Presentation Settings

Most speaking engagements can be broken down into three main types: Formal, semiformal, and informal. Each type shares some common themes with the other categories, yet also contains its own set of recommendations.

Formal

Formal presentations center around organized functions, such as speaking to a board of health on future health promotion endeavors, or presenting at a legislative luncheon. Style of dress should be conservative and neat, being careful not to detract attention from the presentation. Detracting accessories should be kept to a minimum. For example, women should avoid gaudy jewelry, overpowering perfume, and heavy makeup. Similarly, men should avoid strong cologne.

The physical setup of a formal presentation usually includes a podium with the speaker slightly elevated above the crowd on a platform or stage. Audiences tend to be larger, ranging anywhere from 50 to 100 or more individuals. Making a concentrated effort to speak eloquently (although this should be done regardless of the presentation type) reflects a sense of knowledge and confidence with the topic. Classic quotes or the use of polished vocabulary terms increases audience respect for the speaker. Often, much is at stake due to the number of powerful people in attendance. Solid impressions made in formal presentations can garner support and help further your cause.

Semiformal

Examples of semiformal settings include employee in-services, facilitating an educational or behavior change workshop, guest speaking at a school, or conducting a professional conference break-out session. Clothing choices for semiformal presentations tend to be less rigid than in formal situations. For men, dress pants and a sports coat or tie will suffice, while for women, a casual skirt, and a simple shirt or sweater will usually be adequate. When in doubt, however, it is better to dress up a notch. The environment of a semiformal presentation is generally more personable than that of a formal presentation. For example, chairs may be arranged in a circular fashion, or in a U-shape in order to promote group cohesiveness. Group size usually does not exceed 40 or 50 people. Health education jargon (e.g., epidemiological *incidence* and *prevalence, assessment* and *assurance, cardiovascular disease risk reduction strategies*) should be used sparingly so that participants are not confused, intimidated, or uninterested. Given that it is less strict than the formal environment, tasteful humor can be implemented.

Due to its semiformal nature, professionals may underestimate the importance of the speech or program and approach it with less rigorous standards. The same amount of time and energy that is put into preparing a formal presentation should also be expended for a semiformal engagement as well. Word of how well someone is able to convey information travels quickly. It is normally through medium to small presentations that a speaker is recommended for larger, more formal ones. Semiformal, therefore, does not mean half the effort and energy, it means a great opportunity to do more.

Informal

Informal presentations tend to offer the greatest amount of pleasure and the least amount of stress because they involve a much more relaxed atmosphere. Typical informal scenarios might include sharing monthly accomplishments with coworkers at a department meeting, or conducting focus group discussions with seventh and eighth graders. Style of dress should be casual, with the goal to be comfortable without looking careless. Rooms can be set up in any of the previously mentioned ways, and can be changed upon arrival if needed. Group size usually consists of less than 25 individuals. For language style, speakers should stick to the basics, with minimal use of complex vocabulary terms, jargon, or acronyms. Normally a conversational approach to speaking works best, with humor and activities to help the process. Informal presentations can provide a chance for speakers to get to know each member of the audience. Do not, however, let the informal atmosphere be deceiving. Because informal presentations are less rigid, the speaker has tremendous latitude in presentation style. At times, professional skills may slip, and minor, yet important, details are neglected. It is important, then, that informal presentations are given the preparation time that is necessary in order to be effective.

Speakers should always make sure that words on overheads are correctly spelled, handouts are neat, and the organization of material is easy-to-follow for the participants. Regardless of whether the presentation is formal, semiformal, or informal, qualities of effective speakers are universal. Speakers who are considerate, genuine, trustworthy, enthusiastic, and proficient, are more likely to capture and maintain an audience's attention than someone that appears egocentric, uncaring, dishonest, and misinformed (see Table 6-1 for characteristics of effective speakers).

THE PRESENTATION OPENING

Prior to actually starting a presentation, the speaker must first greet the participants. The type of approach will depend on the type of presentation. For instance, the speaker may stand in the doorway greeting participants as they enter the room. In contrast, greeting the audience as a key note speaker at a professional conference may simply involve thanking them for the opportunity to present. When given the opportunity, greet participants with a handshake. It is amazing what impressions are made through a simple handshake. Equally amazing is that many people do not know the proper way to shake someone's hand. Those who have a weak, clammy handshake come across as insecure, uninterested, or rude. Individuals who use a firm grip are seen as more confident, professional, sincere, and attentive. Proper handshaking techniques, as outlined in Table 6-2, can make the difference in building rapport with and respect from participants.

The saying, "You never get a second chance to make a first impression," directly impacts how the speaker should begin the presentation. This is because an audience will draw conclusions about the presenter and the topic within the first few minutes of the session. Therefore, it is very important that speakers carefully plan how to begin. Several techniques, such as humor, relevant stories, and audience questions, can be used.

Humor

Most audiences, regardless of the setting, enjoy humor, especially as an ice breaker. Humor, in fact, may well be one of the greatest assets of a polished

Table 6-1. Characteristics of an Effective Speaker

- *Considerate.* Listening and validating the concerns, opinions, and reactions of participants shows that the speaker values the audience's input as much as their own.

- *Genuine.* Making up information, giving false compliments, or using over dramatic wording can lead the audience to believe that the speaker is only there to be liked.

- *Trustworthy.* Good speakers create trust by being honest and sincere, and using credible sources of information. If the data seems out-of-date or debatable, the audience may ignore what is being said.

- *Enthusiastic.* The excitement that surrounds a speaker that genuinely appears excited about the information being presented is catchy. Enthusiastic presenters maintain audience attention because they convince the audience that the information they are presenting is exciting, interesting, and important.

- *Humorous.* Appropriate humor personalizes the topic and allows the speaker to make light of subjects that can be complex or intense.

- *Proficient in subject.* Being prepared and well-versed in the topic being presented shows dedication and commitment. Having a degree of proficiency in the topic increases credibility and trustworthiness from the audience's perspective.

speaker. People naturally like to laugh and speakers like audience approval that is associated with laughter. In order for humor to be effective, it must be tasteful, applicable, and non-degrading. For example, a joke on how unpredictable teenagers are may not receive an encouraging response from a group of teenagers. They could find it attacking, or an example of someone who "does not understand them." A joke on parent quirks, however, may show a common thread of understanding. Humor does not necessarily mean using jokes. Clever anecdotes or cartoons may be as equally effective. In fact, having a transparency with an applicable cartoon before the program has begun can help the audience understand what will be discussed, while eliciting an initial humorous reaction.

Relevant Stories

In more formal settings, many speakers begin presentations with a relevant news event or short personal story. Before engaging in a program on nutrition, for example, a speaker may recall the struggles of how difficult it was to choose a healthy meal in the cafeteria. Stories express familiarity with the subject from both a professional and a personal perspective which allows for a stronger connection with the audience. When participants find a speaker to be real, they tend to pay more attention throughout the presentation.

Posing Questions to the Audience

Posing a question is an effective way to get attention because it causes the audience to focus their attention on the topic. For instance, "What household accident currently takes the lives of over 8,000 children every year?" makes the audience focus on the topic because it requires a specific response. If using this type of question, time needs to be allowed for a response. In contrast, the question, "How do we stop household accidents from occurring?" does not require a response but requires the audience to ponder the issue. Each of these methods focuses attention in the direction of the topic and includes the mental participation of the audience.

USING EFFECTIVE PRESENTATION SKILLS

Effective presenters are keenly aware of messages the body and voice convey to the target audience. For example, part of understanding the words "Be careful!" comes from a person's movement, tone, and facial expressions. While saying, "Be careful!" and trying to create the impression of a warning, the body moves with a quick jerk, the tone is high and shrieking, and the eyes are wide open. The picture is complete for the audience. These components of communication offer more than just the uttering of sounds. The presenter connects feeling to the sounds, and the feelings help to make for a dynamic program.

With regard to communication skills, it has been found that only 7% of what the audience understands comes from spoken words. The other 93% comes from voice tone and pitch, facial expressions, and mannerisms.[3,4] In essence, the "meaning starts in your mind, flows to your body, then through symbols of gesture, tone and expression flows to your audience."[4] How a message is communicated is just as important as what is said.

Table 6-2. Handshaking Guidelines

What to do
- Extend the arm out, away from the body.
- Hold fingers close together, with thumb up.
- Grip firm enough so that the hand wraps around the person's hand.
- Smile and make eye contact.

What not to do
- Keep arm close at side, only lifting the hand.
- Spread out fingers and thumb.
- Grip so hard that the participant's hand aches.
- Grip loosely with no pressure.
- Frown, scowl, look uninterested, or look away.

Imagine, for example, a presentation on HIV/AIDS. Given the nature of this topic, some educators struggle with their own levels of discomfort and fear. They may stutter, speak with a condescending air, or nervously giggle. To the audience, this could appear that the instructor is uninformed and unprofessional. The presenter may walk away feeling extremely proud of the performance and remain completely oblivious to what really transpired. To avoid this, the presentation should be practiced in front of peers ahead of time. Following the presentation, their impressions of the verbal and nonverbal messages should be discussed. Practice heightens awareness of verbal and nonverbal cues in advance, thus ensuring a positive impression in a real presentation.

Verbal Cues

The manner in which the presenter speaks directly impacts the conclusions an audience makes about the speaker's opinions and beliefs. Because "the voice is a flexible and complicated instrument," the feelings behind words should be considered before they are actually spoken.[1] What a speaker says, and *how* it is said, has a great deal to do with what the speaker is thinking. Presenters need to consider how accurate and clear their message sounds to others. Concise oral communication is valuable because it tends to be the strongest driving force behind the final decision of a person, group, or company.[4]

There are four principal verbal cues: Word accentuation, pitch and tone, pace, and volume. Appropriate use of verbal cues helps the listener connect to the presenter on a deeper level. Characteristics of good presenters include the ability to use vocal variety, emphasize key concepts with inflection, and gain attention through volume.[4]

Word Accentuation
Word accentuation is the process of emphasizing certain words to let the listener know that a word or phrase is particularly important. Effective speakers are able to slow their pace in midstream, without the audience being consciously aware, in order to highlight important words or phrases. Generally, a short pause following an accentuation helps drive the importance of the point. A presentation of the state of the current U.S. health care system can be used to illustrate this point. Accentuating the total cost of health care goods and services in the U.S. (e.g., one *trillion* dollars), emphasizes the seriousness of the problem.

Pitch
Pitch is associated with voice octave and can fluctuate from low to high. Like word accentuation, variation in pitch can be used to emphasize points. For instance, raising and lowering the pitch can create doubtfulness or

uncertainty (e.g., "I *think* so"). Placing a higher pitch at the end of a phrase demonstrates uncertainty or questioning (e.g., "They *are?*"). A lower pitch usually represents endorsement (e.g., "It *can* be done"). Variation in pitch is a useful technique in situations where the speaker wants to elicit emotional reaction or support.

Tone

Tone is the patterns in which a pitch is placed. The main objective with tone is not to follow a chant-like or monotone pace, as this can have a numbing effect on participants. Listening to someone speak monotone, despite how fascinating the topic may be, detracts from maintaining interest levels. When practicing speeches, presenters should get into the habit of recording their voice and listening to it. If there is little variation in pitch and tone, key sentences should be determined in which pitch and tone could be utilized.

Pace

Pace is the acceleration or deceleration of the presentation. It should be varied enough so the audience does not appear to be drifting into a coma (generally this is not a good sign). Sometimes a speaker will slow down the pace of a speech in order to create a sense of intrigue or suspense. Speeding up momentarily could represent an increasing level of excitement. Too much speed, however, could confuse an audience due to lost words and pronunciations. Speakers should watch to make sure that the tempo is comfortable for the audience. A good sign that the pace may be too fast is when members of the audience start to appear confused or irritated, ask if the presenter could repeat what was just said, or begin talking amongst themselves in order to find out what was missed. The presenter should ask the audience if the pace is adequate whenever individuals appear confused or frustrated.

Volume

None of the previously mentioned verbal cues will matter if the presenter is not loud enough. Regardless of where presenting (e.g., a large or small room, outdoors or indoors), voice volume must raise and lower accordingly. The speaker should always ask the audience if the volume is adequate. If not, the speaker should make adjustments rather than asking the audience to "just move closer." Placing that type of responsibility on a participant is rude. It is not the responsibility of the audience to make sure a speaker's volume is satisfactory. It is the *speaker's* job to monitor whether or not the audience can hear by changing their volume until the listeners are accommodated.

Knowing the makeup of the audience beforehand can aide in planning appropriate voice volume. For instance, older populations may have diminished hearing, especially with regard to high pitched and soft-spoken sounds. Appropriate voice volume is also dependent on the room setup and structure. For longer rooms, speakers should "throw" their voice toward the back of the room, so that the sound has a better chance of reaching those sitting near the back. A room that is short in length and wide requires less volume from the speaker, but more turning while speaking to ensure that individuals sitting at both sides of the room can hear. Participants feel left out if they cannot hear the speaker.

Nonverbal Cues

Imagine yourself at a conference listening to the keynote speaker. You notice that the speaker makes little eye contact with the audience and often stares at an oblivious point in space. The speaker stands in one place, slumped over notes. Without even hearing what was said, what impressions do you get? A few years back, my colleagues and I attended a conference where this happened. Our table was horrified, angry, and annoyed as to why someone with such poor speaking skills would be made the keynote speaker. Despite how valuable the information was, we were so distracted with the negative nonverbal cues that we ended up directing our attention elsewhere. Was the speaker nervous? Uninterested in the topic? Or simply unconscious of the real messages being sent? Regardless, it ruined what could have otherwise been a valuable presentation.

Nonverbal cues are those impressions given to a person, group, or audience with facial expressions, body movements, and other gestures. Nonverbals aid the speaker in a smooth presentation delivery by reconfirming the meaning behind a spoken word. The first impression audiences usually pick up from speakers is the way they *appear*, such as standing tall, staring at the ground, or fidgeting with objects. Delivery is just as crucial as presentation content.[2] Important nonverbal cues in presentation delivery include posture, eye contact, body movement, and facial expressions.

Posture

Good posture portrays confidence and expertise. Proper posture necessitates standing tall, with the chest slightly out, and the head back. Presenters that stand with feet shoulder width apart, hands at the waist, and weight concentrated more on the balls of the feet, appear more attentive. Speakers who sit in a chair or hide behind tables or podiums are at a disadvantage because when they start to move around (which all good speakers should do), it appears awkward. Standing center stage without any of the previously described "crutches" make for a strong first impression.

Equally important is the ability to adapt posture to the type of presentation. An erect, stoic posture associated with a formal presentation may be intimidating or awkward for an informal setting. Similarly, resting on a table, which may be appropriate in an informal situation (e.g., facilitating a support group), would be inappropriate in a formal setting. In general, it is better to err on the side of being over professional.

Eye Contact
Lack of eye contact may show distrust, apprehension, nervousness, lack of confidence, trepidation, or boredom. In contrast, appropriate eye contact portrays confidence and connects the speaker with the audience at a personal level. Effective use of eye contact includes connecting briefly (i.e., 1-2 seconds) with different listeners throughout the presentation. The speaker must be careful, however, not to focus on a single individual for an extended period of time. Scanning over people and stopping periodically at random individuals ensures the presenter will not focus too long on one particular person. Whether in a job interview, presenting to a small group of 10-12 individuals, or giving a large lecture, skillful eye contact can be the difference between a great interaction and a mediocre one. It is important to remember that each person in the audience wants to feel like he or she is a part of the presentation. Effective use of eye contact allows this connection to occur.

Body Movement
Body movement is a nonverbal cue that can create different degrees of intimacy, warmth, and friendliness. In addition, speakers who move freely demonstrate a greater level of comfort with themselves and the topic and tend to maintain a higher level of audience interest. For example, arm and hand gestures are wonderful ways to express feelings. Waving the arms and hands about during a comment like "What can we do?" has a greater impact than if it were to be said with the arms resting on a podium or at the speaker's sides. Gestures like pointing or giving the "okay" sign help to clarify or define a point. Body movement is not effective, however, unless the speaker has a purpose behind the movement. Some scripted presenters are choreographed on where and how they should stand, which can appear unnatural. Rather than thinking "At the end of this sentence I will move seven feet to the right," it is better to be in tune with the impact of the words and move according to the rise and fall of emotions. This way, listeners can see and feel the emotions along with the speaker.

Speakers need to be aware of when their movement becomes distracting rather than enhancing. Over use of arm movement can portray hyperactivity or nervousness. Similarly, pacing becomes irritating to listeners who are trying to hear a trailing voice. Effective speaking involves being able to remain in one spot until a natural break occurs in a thought process (e.g., end of a concept), where the speaker can move without disrupting the listeners' flow of information. In general, a speaker should never change positions until a thought has been finished. Similarly, a speaker should never start a new thought until all movement has stopped, and the speaker is firmly positioned. Paying attention to audience reactions is always a helpful cue.

Facial Expressions

Facial expressions can be used to pull the audience towards unspoken insinuations. For example, a lifting of the eyebrows at the tail end of a question may show a desire for a response. Grimacing while reading the latest inoculation rates for infants could be used to show the need for improvement. It is through facial expressions that an audience witnesses the sincerity of a presenter.

Some speakers consistently appear to be unhappy with having to present. Others have a tendency to appear bored. These speakers fail to use one of the most powerful public speaking facial expressionsæa smile. A genuine smile can display warmth, affection, sincerity, or sympathy. As long as the information is not too serious, a smile can go a long way. If there is one surefire way to help win over an audience, it is the speaker who is not afraid to smile.

Every speaker has at least one facial characteristic that is strikingly noticeable during a presentation. For some, it is their smile. Others may have dark, deep-set eyes or expressive eyebrows. Still others may have pronounced forehead lines or a dimple in the cheek. Being aware of this trait can aid the speaker in using facial expressions to accentuate a phrase or concept.

AVOIDING PRESENTATION PITFALLS

In addition to effective presentation skills, speakers should be attentive to negative presentation characteristics that could potentially reduce the impact of the message being presented.

Distracting Mannerisms

In addition to effective verbal and nonverbal cues, it is just as important for a speaker to be aware of distracting verbal and nonverbal mannerisms. For instance, almost every speaker has a favorite "nuisance word" that tends to be inserted between thoughts and during lulls in the presentation. Words such as "um," "okay," "like," "you know," and "ah" are irritating and distracting to the audience. With the overuse of these words, the audience begins to anticipate the next utterance of the nuisance word, drawing attention away from the information being presented. To overcome using these words, the speaker needs to be aware of when a thought finishes, and rather than uttering a sound, keep quiet. At first, the silence that exists seems eternal. This is not all bad though, because the audience sometimes needs a moment to digest what has been said before moving on to the next point. With practice, speakers can train themselves on how to connect thoughts without using a nuisance word.

Another distracting mannerism is fidgeting with one's jewelry, hair, beard, or other distracting item. Most speakers are unaware when they are being distracting. Twisting a finger in their necklace, combing their hands through their hair, or constantly pushing their hair behind their ear can become second nature. Speakers usually are not consciously aware of the distracting mannerisms. The audience, however, becomes keenly aware and irritated with these actions. Practicing in front of a mirror or in front of peers will aid in identifying these mannerisms. In a similar manner, peer review will assist in identifying distracting practices such as placing hands in pockets, jingling coins or keys in pockets, or "massaging" chalk or white board markers. A checklist, similar to that found in Figure 6-1, could be used by peers to identify unwanted mannerisms. Table 6-3 consists of common distracting mannerisms and suggestions for overcoming them.

Figure 6-1. Distracting Mannerisms Checklist

Distracting Mannerism	*Number of Times Observed*	
Nuisance word	_____	Word: _____
Fidgeting with personal item (e.g., hair, tie)	_____	Item: _____
Fidgeting with writing implement	_____	Item: _____
Adjusting clothing, jewelry	_____	
Fixating on ground/back of room	_____	
Pacing	_____	
Hands in pockets	_____	
Arms crossed	_____	
Poor posture	_____	
Low voice volume	_____	
Speed (too fast or slow)	_____	

Table 6-3. Strategies for Overcoming Common Distracting Mannerisms

Mannerism	*Strategy for Overcoming*
Nuisance word	When ending a thought or sentence, be sure to close your mouth and avoid uttering sounds. Practice speaking short unrelated points while focusing on the transition between thoughts or sentences.
Fidgeting with personal item	Use arms and hands during explanations. If hands are part of the presentation, they are less likely to roam and distract the audience. Make a point of being able to see your hands out of the corner of your eye throughout the presentation. Keep pockets empty to avoid the temptation of playing with keys and lose change. When finished writing with board marking pens or chalk, place them on the table so that hands remain free to communicate. Style hair so it stays out of your face and eyes.
Fixating on a point in the back of the room or on the ground; no eye contact	Maintain eye contact with audience members, especially at the start of every new idea.
Pacing	Walk to a pre-designated spot in the room and stay there until the point being made is complete. Be aware of the audience having difficulty in following your movement.

Presentation Sins

In addition to distracting mannerisms, there are many ways in which a presentation can fail. Being attentive to these potential pitfalls increases the likelihood of a successful presentation, which in turn, increases the likelihood that the audience will apply what has been presented.

Some of the more common "sins" that speakers engage in include the following:[3]

- *Apologizing in advance for out-of-date, boring, or ill-prepared material.* Due to the nature of the information, not all presentations bring about the same level of interest. Starting a speech with "I know this stuff is really dull so I will try to be quick about it," is negative and suggests to the audience that the presentation will be boring and useless. Excuses for typed errors, lack of current data, forgotten handouts, or laziness should not be mentioned to the audience. They do not care and it places their mind set in a more critical state. Instead, the speaker should apologize for the lack of preparation and indicate how it will be corrected in the future. Speakers who often find themselves poorly prepared should consider ways to more effectively manage their time.

- *Apologizing in advance for using small writing on overheads.* If the visuals are ineffective, do not use them. It is better to verbally present the information than try to use a distracting, hard-to-read overhead.

- *Being unable to articulate to the audience why the subject is important.* If the speaker cannot think of any reasons to be there, why should the audience? It is the speaker's job to know their "purpose." Furthermore, the speaker must believe in what is being presented. If the speaker does not believe in the message, how can the audience be expected to believe in it?

- *Using the same presentation for different audiences.* Because different audiences have different needs, using the same presentation without updating the materials will likely result in an ineffective presentation. For example, conducting a presentation on nutrition to high school seniors and then delivering the same presentation to a senior citizen group would be inappropriate.

- *Discussing too much information.* Minute details, monotonous tangents, and unnecessary story telling should be left out of presentations altogether. Adhere to the objectives of the presentation and avoid giving unnecessary information that will confuse the audience. The audience will not remember the irrelevant details, but they will remember a speaker who talks too long.

- *Turning the lights out to show a slide show and read a script.* Keep away from script reading at all costs when the lights are out, as it appears unprofessional. Instead, know the material so that it can be paraphrased.

- *Reading every word from every visual.* Try and add other ideas during the presentation that are not displayed on the visual. Also, make sure the visuals are written at an appropriate reading level.

- *Unrehearsed.* Those who do improvisational presentations rarely leave an audience impressed. Practice makes perfect.

- *Failing to start and end on time.* Nothing is more frustrating to an audience than a speaker who is late or runs over the time allotted for the presentation. Be aware of the time both before and during the presentation. If needed, assign a colleague (or room monitor) to serve as a time keeper.

- *Displaying long, heavy sighs.* These show listeners that the speaker is anything but thrilled to be there. Why should the audience feel any different?

THE PRESENTATION CLOSING

The shortest part of the entire presentation is the closing. An effective closing is like placing the final ribbon on a wrapped gift. A poorly formed
ending, however, can erase much of what preceded it. Although most participants will focus on the positive aspects of a presentation, some may
completely fail to remember anything but a weak ending. Effective presentation closings include (1) offering a challenge to the audience, (2) summa-
rizing major points that were presented, and (3) calling on participants to
improve the future by taking action.[5,6]

Audience Challenges

Challenges made to an audience are intended to promote a continued sense
of commitment. They work particularly well in settings where change is
desired. For instance, a group can be challenged to donate at least 10 hours
a month to a volunteer organization, or to lower current rates of heart disease in a community by 15%. Challenges can be used to motivate action.
For instance, Dr. Laura Schlessinger, a popular talk radio personality, ends
her programs by saying, "Now . . . go take on the day!"

Reminders of Past Points

As previously mentioned, the presentation could open with a question or
an anecdote. A great way to help the audience remember key points is to
finish with a summary of answers or a continuation of the anecdote. When
properly planned, a concluding "tie-in" can be powerful. It has the potential for creating many different moods, all of which can lead to a heightened level of awareness as demonstrated in the following story:

> At a seminar focusing on teenage mothers, the speaker began by tell-
> ing a story of a young 14-year old pregnant girl who was surrounded
> by violence and poverty. The body of the presentation focused on a
> new approach to working with pregnant teens in poor areas. Near
> the end of the program, we were reminded of this teen and told about
> her success and the changes that had taken place in her life. As we
> left the room, we felt hopeful and motivated to help pregnant teenag-
> ers.

Call to Action

Action, or a lack of action, has an impact on the future. Therefore, this is an
extremely strong point in closing. It paints a picture of how things *could* be
if the audience attempts some of the recommendations made in the speech.
The ending to a presentation about seat belt safety could be "And so, by

remembering to buckle up, we could reduce the number of fatal accidents by over 30% each year. Life and health insurance rates would slowly decrease and severe injury rates would plummet." The goal of this closing is to inspire individuals to become active participants in their world, health, and future.

THE QUESTION AND ANSWER PERIOD

A question and answer (Q&A) segment following a presentation shows that the presenter is trustworthy and concerned that the audience understood what was presented. The presenter's goal should be to stay as relaxed and in control as possible, while adequately and accurately responding to audience questions. Although Q&A sessions are easier to implement in smaller groups, they should also be included in larger settings. Often a larger gathering has an agenda that indicates time set for a designated Q&A segment.

Speakers can invite participants to ask questions. This demonstrates that the presenter is willing and able to listen to the group. Some participants, however, may be insecure about making an inquiry in front of a large group, or embarrassed with the question they have. In this situation, the speaker may want to politely mention that if there are any questions individuals who would prefer to ask a question in private, they are welcome to do so when the program is finished.

Although question and answer sessions are usually constructive and beneficial to the audience, some presentations will have a select few who, consciously or unconsciously, seek to negatively control the stage. This is especially true with presentations that are controversial such as sex education or environmental issues. These participants demand extra attention for a variety of reasons. The initial response could be to give up authority for fear of confrontation, although this would hinder the speaker's competence. When a loss of authority is sensed by the audience, certain individuals may see the opportunity for a takeover. The remainder of this section describes ways to regain control from three types of participant distracters.

The Debater

The first of these presentation distractions involves the *debater*. The purpose behind debaters' comments are to prove to the audience that the speaker is incompetent, or less knowledgeable than themselves. The debater may sit silently until it is time for questions and answers, or rudely interrupt from the very beginning. When speaking on controversial topics such as contraception, homelessness, sexually transmitted diseases, or homosexuality, a debater is usually present.

The debater should be allowed to speak without interruption. Taking time to understand this person's perspective does not mean an alteration of the presenter's personal viewpoints and convictions. Instead, it is meant to increase tolerance and participation by all audience members. A speaker's attitude of "I am right, you are wrong" only damages the effectiveness of both the presenter and the presentation. Being well informed in advance on different perspectives shows debaters that their opinion is not neglected. An immediate calming effect may take hold when the debater sees that the speaker has no intention of engaging in a heated debate. Validating the debater can occur by using phrases like "I have never thought of it that way, thanks for sharing your opinions with us", or "That is an interesting point." Debaters usually just want to know that they are being heard.

The Expert

Experts are persons, or groups, who feel their level of expertise exceeds that of the speaker. They may preface comments by announcing their credentials and years of experience in order to validate what is about to be said. The following author experience illustrates the expert:

> *Recently I had an encounter with an expert. When presenting a university program on nutrition, I met a gentleman in the audience who was studying to be a Dietitian. Throughout the program, he would interrupt and add comments to my information. Many times he would raise his hand for a question, and instead, would describe personal experiences with nutritional research. I noticed that participation had considerably dropped and people had given up trying to compete with him. I felt I had lost control. By the end of the session, audience members were irritated enough that one actually asked him to be quiet.*

Normally, the expert means well. They are excited about the topic presented because of their personal aptitude and, therefore, tend to be a bit overzealous. Interestingly, many experts have an abundance of useful information that can work to a speaker's advantage. When an expert is given the freedom to interrupt and dominate the conversation, however, the speaker quickly loses credibility. If it so happens that the experts are in fact, *true* experts, they need to be reminded that most of the audience are not experts. They need to be gently persuaded that a need exists for others to participate. If this does not work, an unscheduled break can be taken in order to talk to the expert one-on-one. Explanations like, "You sure do know a lot of information. I have found it very helpful. Could you *silently* critique my information and then we can discuss anything you would like to add or correct when I am finished?" or "Since you are up-to-date on this, I would like to focus my energies on those who are not. I am sure you understand." This can help to alleviate potential problems with experts. The expert should know that this is not a personal attack, but rather a compliment. The presentation needs to be geared towards the majority, and usually the majority of listeners are not experts.

The Poor Listener

Sometimes, individuals who ask the most questions do so because they failed to listen to the information. This can be terribly annoying for a speaker. Characteristics associated with *poor listeners* include the following:

- After just a few sentences, poor listeners decide whether or not a speaker is boring or interesting.

- If a speaker displays unusual characteristics (e.g., wears wild clothing), poor listeners are more likely to be judgmental about the information presented.

- Good organization helps poor listeners to focus better. Poor listeners miss a lot of the presentation's generalizations and interpretations. They find it easier to stick to the hard facts.

There are many ways to reduce the number of poor listeners in a group, including the following:[1]

- Pay special attention to the opening statements made in a speech. Because the poor listener is quickly distracted, ensure the beginning of the presentation has a relevant quote, video segment, or eye catching visual.

- Dress conservative and neat. Ideally, no one should be discriminated against because of appearance, but nevertheless, it does happen. The speaker needs to be remembered for the speech, not (e.g.) the "wild hat" that was worn while presenting.

- The better a presentation is organized, the greater the chances of reaching a higher percentage of audience members. Poor organization can be especially difficult for poor listeners, as jumping from thought to thought can confuse them. Having a structured outline (either as a handout or overhead transparency) to follow while speaking helps to keep everyone on track.

CONCLUSION

Learning the art of exceptional presentation preparation and public speaking is essential for health educators. Public speaking does not always apply to a crowd of people and a podium; it involves a variety of opportunities for sharing health education messages. Regardless of setting, the more proficient the speaker, the more likely the audience will absorb information that will assist them in maintaining their health.

Effective public speaking is a skill that can be learned. In fact, it is a skill that all health educators, regardless of current speaking skills, could and should improve. For many, it will take a great deal of practice and experience, but the benefits far outweigh the costs.

References

1.   Reid, L. (1972). *Speaking well* (2nd ed.). New York: McGraw-Hill.

2.   Whitman, R., J., & Foster, T. J. (1987). *Speaking in public.* New York: McMillan Publishing Company.

3.   Peoples, D. A. (1988). *Presentations plus: David Peoples' proven techniques.* New York: John Wiley & Sons.

4.   Whalen, D. J. (1996). *I see what you mean.* Thousand Oaks, CA: Sage Publications.

5.   Miller, N. E. (1946). Speech introductions and conclusions. *Quarterly Journal of Speech, 32,* 181-183.

6.   Bradley, B. E. (1981). *Fundamentals of speech communication: The credibility of ideas* (3rd ed.). Dubuque, IA: William C. Brown.

Chapter 7

MARKETING AND PUBLIC RELATIONS

Shelly E. Schadewald, M.A., C.H.E.S.
Lisa R. Rutherford, M.A., C.H.E.S.

Authors' Comments: *Marketing and public relations are exciting components of any health educator's position. They not only offer the opportunity to be creative and sell a product, service, or behavior to a target population, but also provide an avenue for learning about a population's needs, behaviors, life-styles, and values.*

With each step in our careers, there have been opportunities to exercise marketing principles and build public relations skills. We have been amazed at how public relations can assist organizations, with markedly different philosophies, collaborate. We have also been intrigued with the remarkable things that can be learned about target populations, such as what attracts kids to healthy messages, through marketing efforts. It is exciting to see the impact of effective marketing and public relations to actually see rates of disease dropping or to be able to measure changing opinions or norms of healthy behavior.

This chapter is designed to provide the reader with tips and guidelines for working through the marketing and public relations process. As you explore marketing and public relations, remember that each experience is an opportunity to learn something new. Therefore, enjoy the process.

INTRODUCTION

Marketing and public relations are key to health education and health promotion because they work together to (1) identify the wants and needs of selected segments of a target audience, (2) create awareness for the program and its purpose, and (3) connect individuals, groups, and communities to health services and healthy behaviors.

Marketing

Marketing of health education issues, programs, and services involves determining what various segments of the target population (also called market segments) want and need and developing programs and services to satisfy those wants and needs.[1] Marketing is the process of planning and executing the development, pricing, promotion, and distribution of goods and services to achieve organizational goals by satisfying consumer wants and needs.[2]

Social marketing is a term commonly used to label marketing practice in health education. It is a process that encompasses several components. These components include, among others:[3]

- *Consumer orientation.* Focusing on the needs and interests of target populations.

- *Audience analysis and segmentation.* The application of qualitative research to gather information on the needs and interests of the target population.

- *Formative research.* Message design and pretesting materials.

- *Marketing mix.* The process of identifying product, price, place, and promotion, known as the "four P's" of marketing.

Social marketing, in particular, is closely linked with health education processes as it centers on (1) promoting a health ideal or behavior, (2) reinforcing other health education programming, (3) changing social norms related to health behaviors, and (4) influencing public officials about health issues. Thus, as opposed to promoting a product, as is done in business marketing, social marketing involves promoting a program, service, or health behavior practice. Examples of social marketing approaches include antismoking campaigns, "Immunize by 2" campaigns, and the "I'm Worth Waiting For" sexual abstinence commercials produced by the Arthur DeMoss Foundation.

In general, making changes in knowledge are the easiest to make in the social marketing domain. Changing action, behavior, attitudes and values become progressively more difficult to influence.[2] Successful marketing, therefore, looks for existing values and fine tunes programs and messages to meet those values.[4]

Public Relations

Public relations is one aspect of the larger concept of marketing. It is the process of "creating or changing the attitudes, beliefs and perceptions of people by influencing them—primarily with information disseminated through the media."[5] Specific to health education, public relations involves increasing consumer awareness and improving opinions of health issues, programs, services, and agencies. Public relations promotes the positive aspects of a program or an organization to specific audiences.

Among the most common strategies involved in public relations are (1) the timely and appropriate placement of stories, articles, opinion editorial pieces and letters to the editor in newspapers and magazines, and (2) television and radio news interviews with program or agency spokespersons. Public relations can also involve other promotional tactics, ranging from booklets and pamphlets to public presentations, special events, incentives and word-of-mouth communication.[4]

Many organizations select an individual to coordinate public relations activities. This enables all media inquiries to be directed to one person who can establish good working relationships through regular media contact.[1] While other organizational representatives, such as program staff and agency administrators, may be interviewed for public relations opportunities, the public relations contact is always notified and involved to coordinate consistent messages and images of the program or agency.

The Four P's: The Nuts and Bolts to Understanding the Marketing Process

In basic marketing theory, there are four components to the marketing mix commonly called the "four P's," which constitute the greatest portion of the marketing strategy. The marketing mix's components are product, price, place, and promotion.

Product
Anything that can be offered to a market that may meet a want or need.[6] Services, programs, behavioral practices, and health messages are just a few examples of potential health education products.

Price
What consumers pay, or perceive they are paying, for the product. Price can be in terms of monetary cost paid by the consumer, such as the cost of a nicotine patch or the cost of joining a health club. More commonly in the health field, costs will be psychological, physiological, or social in nature. Examples of these types of costs to an individual may include the amount of time to be invested in the behavior change, or physiological symptoms of nicotine withdrawal such as increased hunger and fatigue.

With regard to price, consumers weigh the perceived benefits against the perceived costs of the product. The perceived benefits must outweigh the perceived costs in order for the consumer to value the product. Costs and benefits associated with the program or service need to be considered during program and service development and when designing marketing strategies. What will consumers gain from the program that will be of value to them? What are the costs? Will the gains outweigh the costs of engaging in the behavior?

Costs need to be defined in terms of the price consumers will pay in order to receive the perceived benefits of the service. It is important not to let professional knowledge cloud what is of value to the consumer. For example, the health benefits of not drinking or wearing a seat belt are obvious to a health professional. Many individuals are likely to value their health, but do not see how the benefit of not drinking or wearing a seat belt outweigh the costs. Focus groups are an excellent tool for determining perceived costs and benefits (see Chapter 3, "Conducting Focus Groups").

To take the concept a step further, the principle of exchange (weighing the costs against the benefits) can be linked to health education theory to better illustrate other considerations an individual may go through before acquiring the product. The Health Belief Model hypothesizes that health-related action depends upon (1) the sufficient motivation (benefits) to make the health issue relevant to the consumer, (2) the belief that one is susceptible to the health issue (perceived threat), and (3) the belief that following a specified health recommendation would be useful in reducing or eliminating the perceived threat at an agreeable cost.[7]

Therefore, in order for action to take place, the benefits of overcoming the perceived threat must be great enough to motivate individuals into following a recommended course of action. They must believe the action will reduce or eliminate the threat at an acceptable cost in order to follow through with the action. The weighing of these variables is the "principle of exchange." In order for the consumer to use a product, the benefits must outweigh the costs.

Place

The setting where the service, program or behavior change takes place. In health education, common examples of setting include worksite, community, schools, homes, churches and health care settings.[6] Settings need to be accessible to the target population. For instance, a local school could be an avenue for reaching not only children, but the parents and other family members of the child.

Promotion

Publicity that the product receives is promotion, and can be closely linked with public relations activities. Promotional tools and strategies are the methods used to inform the target population or market segment about the product. There are many examples of promotional tools that may be used to effectively promote the product (see Table 7-1).

The unique combination of product, price, place and promotion selected to reach a market segment is known as the marketing mix. The marketing mix may differ significantly for the same product depending upon the various market segments that need to be reached. The following section further illustrates the variables that go into determining the marketing mix for a market segment, and provides more detail about execution of the marketing plan.

Table 7-1. Promotion Strategies

- pamphlets
- posters
- paycheck stuffers
- incentives
- promotional contests
- public service announcements
- paid advertising (print or air)
- press releases
- special events
- editorials

STEPS TO MARKETING AND PUBLICIZING HEALTH

In order for a marketing or public relations campaign to be successful, a number of steps can be followed that increase the likelihood that campaign goals will be reached. Each of the steps work together to help the campaign succeed. The strength of one step does not necessarily make up for a weakness in another. Equal attention and consideration need to be given to each phase in the development of a marketing or public relations campaign.

The following steps are essential to marketing and publicizing health:[8]

1. Knowing the health issue.

2. Researching the target audience.

3. Identifying the best channel for marketing the message.

4. Pilot testing with a smaller target audience.

5. Fully implementing and continually refining the marketing strategy.

6. Utilizing public relations techniques.

Knowing the Issue

Before undertaking marketing efforts, the health educator must have a clear understanding of the (1) issues and (2) programs and services that are designed to address the issues. If a health educator has been assigned to market programs or services in a particular topic area (e.g., tobacco, abstinence, worksite wellness programs), familiarity and experience with the program or service is critical to understanding all aspects of the product being marketed. If a health educator is in the role of marketing programs and services for which they are not intimately involved, a thorough orientation and regular contact with the program staff are essential to understanding the philosophy, program operations, and controversial aspects of the product before embarking on a marketing initiative.

For example, if a health educator is asked to market the Women, Infants and Children (WIC) program for a local health department, it may be beneficial for the health educator to act as a client for a day and proceed through the certification and educational procedures that clients experience. In addition, spending time with various WIC program staff learning the diverse components of the program will provide additional insight. At any rate, obtaining input from administrators, program staff, clients, and members of the target audience is crucial to developing the marketing approach. The perspectives of each of these groups will provide different and valuable perspectives on the program components and on marketing strategies.

Researching the Target Audience

Central to successful marketing efforts is understanding the characteristics and values associated with desired target audiences that tend to drive adopting healthy behaviors. Many techniques can assist in the identification of target audience characteristics including those presented in Chapters 1 (community assessment), 3 (focus groups), and 14 (diversity). Available sources include community assessment data, health and vital statistics, surveys, focus groups, other health program data, local universities, published research, television and radio stations, and statewide or community-based organizations that work with the target population.

Audience segmentation is the process of identifying the variables that impact target group decision making.[9] Central to this process is the premise that within target audiences there exist segments of the population that have distinct characteristics and values. Strategies must be tailored to each segment in order to be truly effective.

In health education, audience segmentation variables generally include traditional demographic and geographic characteristics whereas in marketing segmentation, psychographic and behavioristic variables are used as well. Psychographic and behavioristic variables are often overlooked in health education (see Table 7-2).[2]

The application of psychographic variables to health education message consideration can be illustrated through an examination of a community health assessment research project conducted by a tri-county consortium of local health departments and a regional community mental health-

Table 7-2. Comparison of Traditional Health Education and Marketing
Segmentation Variables

Health Education Segmentation Variables

Geographic	*Demographic*
• region	• age
• county	• religion
• city	• gender
• neighborhood	• race/ethnicity
• population density	• income
	• education
	• family size

Marketing Segmentation Variables

Psychographic	*Behavioristic*
• social class	• benefits sought
• life-style	• use rates
• personality	• readiness stage
• values	• attitude toward
• opinions	product
• attitudes	

provider. The consortium conducted a three-phase qualitative and quantitative research project as part of a local community health assessment initiative. Building on findings from the qualitative phases (key informant interviews and focus groups) it was quantified through a random sample telephone survey that 92% of respondents had attempted a life-style behavior change in the previous 12 months.[10] The second leading source of support for behavior change (behind "not being able to stand it anymore") was identified as the encouragement of family and friends, with 34.5% of respondents identifying this support as either somewhat or very influential in their behavior change. This suggests that perhaps rather than developing behavior change messages aimed only at the individual, directing messages aimed at family members and friends to encourage a loved one to make a behavior change may be beneficial. It also implies that behavior change messages could be marketed successfully with an emphasis on "do it for someone you love, if not for yourself." These types of messages may be more appealing and effective to large segments of a given target audience.

Identifying the Best Channel for Marketing the Message

Central to developing the marketing plan is identifying the channel for distributing the product to the consumer. Common avenues for promotion include mass media and educational materials such as television, radio, billboards, posters, newspapers, flyers, and brochures. For example, children spend an average of four to five hours per day watching television. Therefore, television can be an excellent avenue for reaching children with social marketing around issues such as nutrition and smoking.

Health information is now advertised on all forms of mass media, in paycheck stuffers, on telephone bills, in newspaper flyers and articles, on cereal boxes, on the Internet, in mall kiosks, and on promotional items like pencils, T-shirts, shoes, and bumper stickers. For example, many cereal boxes now include messages about nutrition and exercise. Worksite wellness programs may be promoted, and employee participation encouraged, through paycheck stuffers. After a worksite wellness program is completed, additional paycheck stuffers may be distributed to employees which include health messages surrounding the reduction of the most significant health risks identified overall among employees.

The approach used to promote the program or service must be persuasive.[8] The consumer must understand, and be at least somewhat convinced, that taking on the healthy behavior that is being promoted is more beneficial (i.e., more valuable on *their* terms) than the previous behavior. A solid understanding of the target audience becomes the mechanism for selecting the marketing strategy best suited to depict that the benefits outweigh the costs.

Pilot Testing

It is necessary to pilot test the marketing plan once it has been developed. Most marketing strategies can be refined or improved as a result of being tested with a sample of the target audience. During pilot testing, samples of materials and suggested messages are presented to members of market segments within the target audience. Feedback is received on different aspects of the proposed marketing campaign before final decisions are made on the materials and marketing strategies.

Focus groups are one commonly used method for pilot testing proposed marketing strategies. For example, participants in the focus group may be presented with proposed materials and strategies for marketing the product. Participants can be asked, through a series of guided questions, for opinions on the effectiveness of the materials. Focus group members may also be asked to identify specifically what aspects of the marketing approach they like or dislike, ranging from the message itself to the spokesperson delivering the message.

The most effective avenues for marketing the product can be identified, through pilot testing, whether it be billboards, radio announcements, personal contacts, or other channels. Specifically, stations and times for airing of advertisements or public service announcements, for example, can be solicited. Even if opinions of market segment representatives are sought prior to development of the marketing campaign, it is important to pilot test the actual marketing tools to determine if the market connects to the message, the promotional tools, and, ultimately, to the product.

Fully Implementing and Refining the Marketing Strategy

Implementation of the marketing plan requires organization, coordination, and attention to detail. Coordinating and scheduling media activities as much as possible in advance will help ensure that the target audience receives messages through various channels over a defined period of time.

Monitoring ensures marketing strategies are targeting the correct audience at the best time, with the most "bang for the buck." Evaluation can help determine the cost effectiveness of given aspects of the campaign, and to determine if the campaign is having the intended effect.

For example, if billboards are produced as part of the marketing campaign, the billboard may include a telephone number people can contact for further information. A tracking sheet can be used to identify the number of calls received in response to seeing the billboard. If after a four-week, $5,000 billboard campaign, only a few calls were received, it would be important to reconsider the cost effectiveness of the campaign and to implement alternative strategies for reaching the target audience. This type of formative evaluation can reveal positive and negative aspects of the campaign, and allow for the development of more appropriate and more effective messages, promotional tools, and marketing strategies.

Public Relations Techniques

As the marketing campaign unfolds, public relations techniques can be implemented to increase awareness and promote a positive image surrounding the campaign. The public relations aspect of the marketing plan acts to build further support for the product being marketed. Public relations must play an important role in marketing efforts as programs are implemented in order to be sensitive to consumers' needs and desires, and also to keep the program protected from negative forces, such as funding shortages or from becoming political footballs, as sometimes happens with sensitive health issues like sex education.

There are several basic steps to effectively utilizing public relations:

1. Prepare press releases, and other appropriate materials to create awareness about the purpose, scope, and applicability of the program or issue. Do not neglect smaller sources such as newsletters or small flyers (e.g., a school PTA newsletter), as well as newspapers, radio, and television.

2. Establish a spokesperson for the program. A spokesperson might be a health educator, supervisor, agency director, or a person of some prominence in the community. Make certain the spokesperson has time and availability for interviews or photo opportunities.

3. Prepare the spokesperson for interviews or "cold calls" from the media by conducting mock interviews. Focus on appropriate and effective body language. Make sure the spokesperson knows the subject matter well and is prepared for additional questions or further clarification.

4. Prepare a list of "difficult" questions that may be asked about the program. Be prepared for negative issues, such as cost, funding sources, program effectiveness. Demonstrate that the program has no hidden agenda. Have a clear purpose prior to implementing any program or marketing strategy.

5. As the program is implemented, solicit news stories or photo opportunities. Track anecdotal information about successes. Implement evaluation strategies throughout program implementation. Both evaluation data and anecdotal information are helpful in fund-raising.

6. Collaborate with other existing events or programs that may coincide with the program, service, or issue being marketed. For example, during *Teen Pregnancy Prevention Month* (May), information about a sex education project could be released to capitalize locally on the national attention being drawn to the issue during that time.

TIPS AND TECHNIQUES FOR SUCCESS

The Power of Persuasion

Often, peer groups have the most influence in persuading a target population to change their behavior or utilize a program. People tend to be persuaded by those with whom they can identify or perceive to be similar to themselves in terms of age, values, or interests. For instance, if children who believe they will benefit from waiting to have sex until adulthood or marriage are supported by their peers, they are more likely to succeed in adopting or changing a certain behavior. In light of this, positive peer pressure techniques and refusal skills are commonly included in many curricula emphasizing healthy behavior.

Establishing Key Indicators to Measure Success

As the marketing plan is being conducted, it is important to evaluate whether the marketing process is being followed and to monitor the marketing plan for necessary adjustments. Questions to ask while the campaign is in place include:

- Is the target audience being reached? Are the numbers of the target audience that was expected to be reached actually receiving the message?

- Is the marketing plan being implemented as planned? Are radio spots, for example, being played with the frequency and during the times specified in the marketing plan?

- What type of feedback has been received regarding the effectiveness of the campaign strategies? What are responses from focus groups, consumer surveys, and interviews? What other feedback has been received from word-of-mouth contact or through phone calls?

- Can people recall the message? Do those contacted through focus groups, consumer surveys, and interviews feel the message is effective?

Being Creative and Utilizing a Diverse Approach

It is essential to revise all tools when necessary, be creative, and use a variety of marketing strategies. Changing strategies at intervals will keep the campaign "fresh." For example, using advertising or public service announcements at certain times that best reach the target audience can easily be switched to a print campaign.[4] This will assist in drawing attention to the issue from those in the target audience who may have not been reached through a different channel. This will also help stretch dollars and maintain variety.

Sensitivity to "Hot" Topics

Caution needs to be taken with sensitive issues such as sex education and child abuse. Due to the controversial nature of sensitive issues, it is important to be prepared to address concerns from the opposition. Looking from all perspectives will increase the likelihood of recognizing potential sticking points. Inviting those with opposing viewpoints into the planning stages of the marketing campaign can help identify potentially controversial aspects of the message, or of certain campaign elements. Strategies for dealing with those issues should then be developed.

For example, in the development of an HIV prevention campaign for teens, it would be critical to invite teens who are representative of the target audience into the marketing campaign planning. Parents of teens, and others who can be identified as potential opponents to the campaign, should also be included. If potential non-supporters are involved in the planning, the opposition may lessen as they gain an increased understanding of the issue, the target audience, and the goals of the marketing campaign. They also may be persuaded once they hear from members of the target audience as to what they believe will be effective.

Empowering the Community

The marketing strategy should empower the community to take action. Individuals need more than information. They need persuasion and support to carry through with healthy behaviors. Cueing individuals to take action to change a behavior and providing information on how to make changes and where to go to find help, are a few simple examples that can help empower individuals to respond actively to the marketing message.

STRATEGIES FOR OVERCOMING BARRIERS

As with any health education strategy, marketing and public relations are not without their share of barriers to implementation. Budget constraints, resistance to the marketing concept (particularly in government agencies) and changing priorities are a few examples of common barriers faced when marketing health education messages, programs, and services. The following tips may help overcome some of the more common pitfalls and barriers involved in marketing health education messages and programs.

Limited Budget

One of the initial barriers for most marketing efforts is a limited budget. Budgets are almost always an unfortunate constraint for marketing programs. A reasonable percentage of the total program budget (10-15%) should be allotted for marketing. Funds should not be wasted on ineffective strategies such as flyers that are not appealing to the target population. Fortunately, there are many marketing strategies, some being low cost, that can be used to market the program or service. Many public relations activities can be carried out at a low cost, and are excellent means to gain publicity and increase awareness. Free avenues for publicity should be used whenever possible.

Establishing positive relationships with local media may increase the likelihood they would assist the effort by serving on committees or coalitions. Media contacts may also be able to devote substantial press coverage to the issue. They may also be able to arrange free or reduced cost air time for the issue.

Organizations may be interested in sponsoring specific requests if they can also benefit from the publicity. It is important to tune into the public relations needs of businesses and community groups when thinking about public relations needs relative to the health message, program, or service that needs to be marketed. In Michigan, for example, McDonald's restaurants became a partner in the state's infant immunization campaign. Special bags and place mats were printed to promote immunizations, and stuffers containing immunization schedules were placed into every customer's bag during the month of April (Infant Immunization Month). Not only was this a good public relations opportunity for McDonald's, but it was also a creative way to increase awareness on immunization issues to parents of young children who no doubt patronize the fast-food chain.

Donations can be solicited, including creative work on advertisements and radio promotions. Linking with other campaigns will save resources and allow for sharing publicity and marketing strategies.

Misreading the Target Audience

A second barrier is not properly researching a target audience, which may be due to lack of time or other resources. A lack of awareness of the target population usually results in program failure because the program or message never reaches the intended audience. With programs that fail, reanalysis of the target audience may uncover changes that are needed to improve success.

Legitimization of Marketing

Some agencies are still reluctant to engage in marketing of health programs, services, or issues, especially if the topic is sensitive.[4] Again, it is important that evaluation and public relations are used throughout implementation in order to convince skeptics about marketing program purpose and importance.

Getting Necessary Technical Assistance

Other health educators and agencies may have access to existing marketing and public relations plans or campaigns. It is recommended to seek out successfully marketed programs and ask if strategies could be shared. For example, individuals who prepared a statewide HIV prevention campaign may be able to share strategies and techniques used in campaign development which would be beneficial at the local level.

"Pro bono" assistance can be sought from local public relations or communications businesses. Much can be learned from previous research. Reading the literature on marketing and social marketing will provide insight into essentials associated with effective strategies and campaigns.

Changing Environments/Priorities

It is important to document anecdotal information and indicators of success in order to survive in changing environments, such as in the decentralization of government and local bureaucracies. A thorough process and program evaluation can provide the needed documentation of progress and success. Collecting anecdotal information, such as testimonials from those affected by a program or service, can speak volumes above other more traditional measures of evaluation. Gathering evidence that a program or service works, in both qualitative and quantitative form, can be a great support in unstable or dynamic environments. Being prepared to defend the program by being armed with evidence of its success, will increase the likelihood of survival.

EXPECTED OUTCOMES

The expected outcomes in a marketing or public relations campaign depend upon the goals of the campaign. If the overall goals of a marketing campaign are to increase the use of a particular health service (e.g., increase the use of breast and cervical cancer screening services among Hispanic women over age 40), then the expected outcomes may tie into the increased use of the service by women in the target audience who are exposed to the marketing message. In a public relations campaign, the goal might be to increase positive perceptions of a service (e.g., improve attitudes and perceptions about breast and cervical cancer screening among Hispanic women over age 40). This could be demonstrated by a change in attitudes about breast and cervical cancer screening among the target audience after the public relations campaign has been implemented. Regardless, one thing is for certain: If, as a result of the campaign, the target audience experienced change in relation to the program goals, the campaign was successful.

In either example, it is implied that data will be collected prior to the campaign initiation so that effects of the campaign can be measured both during its implementation and after its conclusion. This allows for evaluation of the effectiveness that the campaign had on influencing the target audience. If a campaign does not produce the desired outcomes, the evaluation should provide insight as to why so that the program, or the campaign strategies, can be modified as necessary.

CONCLUSION

Marketing and public relations are an important part of planning and implementing a successful health-related program or service and of promoting a health issue. Creativity and attention to detail are essential to the process and, although it takes considerable time and effort, the results (e.g., improved health, changing a social norm) will outweigh the costs for the health educator.

Programs often fail because they are not suited to the target audience's wants and needs. Services may be underutilized because people do not know about the program or how to access it. Marketing and public relations work together to define what is in demand by the target audience and how to best meet that demand.

References

1. Breckon, D. J., Harvey, J. R., & Lancaster, R. B. (1994). *Community health education: Settings, roles, and skills for the 21st century* (3rd ed.). Gaithersburg, MD: Aspen Publication.

2. Denard-Goldman, K. (1997). Panacea, plague or placebo: Marketing's role in meeting community needs. Paper presented at the Great Lakes Chapter of the Society for Public Health Education Mid-Year Conference, April 11, Frankenmuth, MI.

3. Lefebvre, R. C., & Flora, J. A. (1988). Social marketing and public health intervention. *Health Education Quarterly, 15,* 299-315.

4. Manoff, R., & Novelli, W. (1988). Social marketing: Accepting the challenge in public health. Paper presented at the Third Annual National Chronic Disease Prevention and Control Conference, September 20-23, Denver.

5. Mallory, C. (1989). *Publicity power: A practical guide to effective promotion.* Los Altos, CA: Crisp Publications.

6. Wilson, M. G., & Olds, R. S. (1991). Application of the marketing mix to health promotion marketing. *Journal of Health Education, 22,* 254-259.

7. McKenzie, J. F., & Jurs, J. L. (1993). *Planning, implementing and evaluating health promotion programs: A primer.* New York: MacMillan Publishing Company.

8. Smith, W. A., (1993). *The future of social marketing.* Paper presented at the Marketing Conference on Creating Successful Partnerships, American Marketing Association, Ontario, Canada.

9. Meyer, G., & Dearing, J. W. (1996). Respecifying the social marketing model for unique population groups. *Social Marketing Quarterly,* Winter, 44-52.

10. Capital Area Health Alliance. (1997). *Community perceptions of health and health care in the capital area community.* Lansing, MI.

Chapter 8

MEDIA ADVOCACY

Beverly A. Riley, M.A.

Author's Comments: *Media advocacy is exciting because it provides a chance to be involved in public attitude and policy changes. In my field of tobacco control, we have seen an incredible shift in attitude about smoking in public. Much of this is due to information on the toxicity of secondhand smoke, the media regarding health effects associated with smoking, and the emergence of nonsmokers' rights. Media coverage and public opinion have certainly helped to contribute to the number of smoke-free worksites, restaurants, and public places by influencing voluntary policy changes, local ordinances, and state and federal laws. As a result, we have seen a decrease in adult tobacco use in communities and states (e.g., California and Utah) that have policies restricting public smoking. The potential benefits of well-planned media advocacy campaigns are endless.*

    This chapter will help you develop skills and learn "tricks of the trade" for effectively working with the media. It took me approximately six months to shift my thinking from using the media as solely a public information vehicle to developing an advocacy spin on media pieces (e.g., articles, press releases, and interview sound bites). Media advocacy has become second nature to me, and I find it difficult to look at an issue or topic, whether health related or not, without thinking about how to "frame" the issue so that it influences decision makers or the general public. By learning the skills presented in this chapter and sharing what you have learned with others, you are "planting the seeds" for impacting the health of your community.

INTRODUCTION

Media advocacy is the strategic use of mass media to advance public policy by applying pressure to policy makers.[1] The use of media advocacy has evolved as the definition of health problems has shifted from the individual level to the policy level. The traditional use of media by health education practitioners has been to change individual behavior. In contrast, media advocacy involves the use of the media to change public opinion and policy regarding health issues and concerns. What distinguishes media advocacy from traditional health promotion and educational efforts is the outcome of the effort (see Figure 8-1).

Figure 8-1. Traditional Health Education vs. Media Advocacy

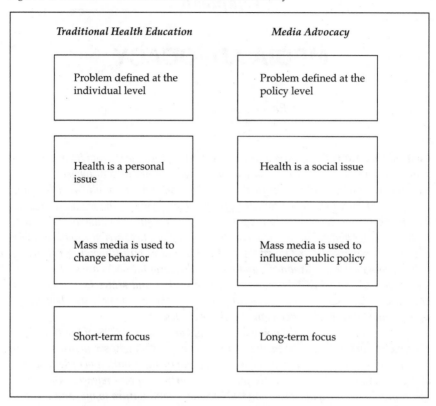

Traditional Health Education	Media Advocacy
Problem defined at the individual level	Problem defined at the policy level
Health is a personal issue	Health is a social issue
Mass media is used to change behavior	Mass media is used to influence public policy
Short-term focus	Long-term focus

An example of this shifting focus can be found in tobacco prevention and control. The problem definition of tobacco use at the individual level is that smoking kills. Youth are taught about the harm of smoking and encouraged not to start, and smokers are encouraged to quit. While these messages are still important for reducing tobacco use, the shift to defining tobacco use as a problem at the policy level leads to broader implications for prevention and behavior change. Instead of "smoking kills," the message becomes "tobacco products kill and it is important to keep them out of the hands of youth." Associated policy changes would include passing stronger laws to prevent the sale of tobacco to youth, licensing of stores and other vendors that sell tobacco, and restricting advertising and promotion of tobacco products to youth.

Media advocacy is a tool that can be used to effectively influence public health policy. The California *Dangerous Promises* alcohol advertising campaign is an excellent example of how media advocacy can successfully alter policy.[1] The premise of the campaign was that alcohol advertising that uses sexist images helps foster an environment where women are less likely to be taken seriously and more likely to be subjected to a range of abusive behaviors. The *Dangerous Promises* campaign's policy goal was to have alcohol advertisers include restrictive guidelines for the depiction of women and themes of sex and violence in their voluntary advertising code of ethics. The initial response of distilled spirit makers was to reject the request to amend their advertising code. After six months of media coverage, which included controversial counter-advertising on billboards, talk radio appearances and interviews with journalists, the distilled spirit makers association adopted two of the three points of the campaign.

STEPS TO CONDUCTING A MEDIA ADVOCACY CAMPAIGN

Avenues for mass media are plentiful in communities, whether in the form of daily or weekly newspapers, television and cable systems, radio stations that target specific audiences, or billboards in neighborhoods and along highways. Faced with a number of different media opportunities available and a variety of messages, it is often difficult to identify where to begin an advocacy approach. Steps for planning and implementing a media advocacy campaign include (1) identifying a policy goal, (2) identifying target audiences that can influence the policy goal, and (3) developing and implementing media strategies.

Identifying a Policy Goal

Because the primary focus of media advocacy is on policy change rather than individual behavior, it is important to first identify a policy goal that will change the community environment. Policies can take many forms, such as legislative (public), organizational (worksite), or procedural (guidelines). For instance, a policy goal might be to pass a local ordinance to restrict placement of billboards advertising tobacco products near schools and playgrounds.

Identifying Target Audiences

Once a policy goal has been determined, those who can make the goal a reality must be identified. Individuals and groups that can influence the policy include local elected officials, parent groups, youth, and the general public. Identifying the various individuals or groups that are influential in setting policy in the community will help determine the most appropriate approach for the advocacy message.

With the *Dangerous Promises* campaign, organizers chose billboard locations close to local television stations to increase the likelihood that reporters would cover the story. The campaign's target audience was not the general public, but rather the leaders of alcohol associations. Campaign organizers believed that adverse media coverage would exert pressure on the alcohol association leadership to change their advertising codes, which would be more effective than pressure from individuals whose awareness had been heightened by the billboards.[1]

There are basically three target audiences for media advocacy: (1) The people with the power to make the policy change, (2) groups or individuals who can wield influence on policy makers, and (3) the general public.[2] For example, the city council has the authority to enact a local ordinance restricting the placement of billboards advertising tobacco products near schools and playgrounds. Neighbors, friends, and constituents can contact members of the city council and express support for such a local ordinance. The general public needs to understand the influence advertising has on youth and tobacco use so they can support a local ordinance.

In addition to key players, it is important to identify other community groups (e.g., PTA, youth groups) that are concerned about the issue and will carry the message forward. What information do these groups need in order to effectively communicate the message to local media? What is the best approach for supplying these advocacy groups with data? Conducting focus groups and public opinion polls can determine what specific groups think about public health problems in terms of causes and solutions (See Chapter 3 "Conducting Focus Groups").[2] The information gleaned in this manner can help advocates deliver the message that is most effective for reaching policy makers.

Direct exposure to the public health problem can build strong alliances with community groups. For example, in promoting an ordinance restricting placement of tobacco advertising, a billboard-mapping project would identify the placement of billboards advertising tobacco products in proximity to schools and playgrounds. Parents, youth, members of the media, and other supportive groups could walk a half-mile radius from schools and count the number of billboards, noting the percentage that advertise tobacco products. Data collected from this mapping strategy can then be shared with individuals and groups to support advocacy efforts.

Developing and Implementing Media Strategies

Central to the success of the advocacy campaign is being able to identify the appropriate media outlets for communicating the advocacy message to the target audience. Becoming a student of the media is critical to the success of the media advocacy campaign. It is important to read daily newspapers, watch local news broadcasts, listen to a variety of radio stations, and be aware of other major media outlets, especially those to which the target audience pays attention.

A number of mechanisms for accessing the media exist. One method is to create news. For instance, following a billboard-mapping project, a press conference can be held at which youth and adults that were involved share the results of their research. Press releases, emphasizing the importance of restricting placement of billboards advertising tobacco products, could be sent to local media outlets. Letters to the editor can conceptualize results of the billboard mapping. A radio news or talk show provides a forum for discussing the results. Relationships can be cultivated with reporters who cover politics and health and youth issues in the community.

Other media avenues include newspapers and other print, electronic media, and paid advertising. Which avenues to use depend on the target audience that is trying to be reached.

Newspaper

Local newspapers, especially the editorial pages, are prime outlets for media advocacy. Editorial pages provide a snapshot of the attitudes and values of a community and are usually read by key community leaders, decision makers, and local elected officials. In addition, they are often tracked by state and federal elected officials. Editorial pages consist of three components: (1) Letters to the editor, (2) opinion editorials (op-eds), and (3) editorials. Letters to the editor and op-eds are written and submitted to the newspaper by community members in response to a newspaper article, another letter to the editor, community issues, or an editorial that has been recently published in the newspaper. Editorials are either written by the newspaper's editorial staff or syndicated.

Letters to the editor provide a glimpse of issues important to the community at any moment in time and often serve to educate and shape the opinions of people in the community. These are the easiest to write and get published. The editorial page usually includes information on how to write a letter to the editor, including the address, word limit, content, and other format guidelines. Following guidelines increases the likelihood of the letter being published.

A letter to the editor offers the rare instance to tell a story without it being interpreted or given a different slant by a reporter. It should include author information (i.e., name, address, and daytime phone number) and be brief (less than 125 words), to the point, in reference to a recent news article, and timely (see Figure 8-2 for a sample letter to the editor).

Signing and spacing submission of letters a few days apart will increase the likelihood of being printed. Papers are not always able to print every letter to the editor, but may be more likely to print similar letters received over a period of time.

Figure 8-2. Sample Letter to the Editor

Letters to the Editor
100 Main Street
Mt. Pleasant, MI 48858

Dear Editor,

The recent admission by the Liggett Company that "the industry markets cigarettes to teenagers" ("Cigarette Maker Owns Up To Addiction," 3/21/97) supports
the importance of restricting billboard advertising in Mt. Pleasant. I believe we
should have a local ordinance that bans billboards that advertise tobacco products
within the city limits. As a parent, it is my responsibility to talk with my children
about the dangers of tobacco use. But I have no control over the larger-than-life
images of people and camels having fun with cigarettes, or spit tobacco that my
children see from the school bus window every morning and afternoon. I need
help from the City Council to eliminate these messages that bombard my children.

Sincerely,

Jane Doe
134 Broadway Street
Mt. Pleasant, MI 48858
773-5238 (daytime phone)

Op-eds are written by citizens in response to a letter to the editor,
editorial, or recent news article. They serve to (1) provide the opportunity
to increase public awareness of an issue, (2) educate policy makers on an
issue, and (3) educate newspaper staff about an issue. Op-eds can influence policy makers by demonstrating growing public awareness and support for a given policy initiative.[3]

Op-eds are longer than letters to the editor, with an average length
of 750 words. Guidelines for op-eds are usually listed on the editorial pages
of newspapers or can be acquired by directly calling the newspaper. A community leader, well-respected health care professional, or parent who has
taken on the role as champion of the advocacy issue, should write the op-
ed. Local media are likely to be more responsive to a local community
member than someone from another city or state.

The op-ed should include a suggested title, the author's name, and a
sentence describing the author's expertise. Contacting the newspaper about
their preferred format and the estimated length of time before publication
will determine if it would be worthwhile to invest the 10-20 hours needed
to write the op-ed.[3] If competition for op-ed space exists, it could be short-
ened and submitted as a letter to the editor. Publication of the op-ed usually appears two weeks after submission.

The op-ed should begin with a few sentences illustrating how the issue affects an individual or group. This will help gain the reader's interest in the piece. Jargon, acronyms, or technical language that would confuse readers should not be used.

Editorials are written by the newspaper's editorial staff. Influencing the editorial board to write a supportive editorial takes thought and planning and is more complicated than submitting a letter to the editor or an op-ed. In essence, the newspaper is being asked to take a stand on a potentially controversial issue in the community. There is a possibility, however, that the newspaper is not supportive and may actually publish an editorial that is in opposition to the media advocacy policy goal.

To increase the likelihood that the editorial board will consider supporting the issue, it is first important to discover positions the paper has previously taken on the issue. How long ago was the editorial? Was the position taken by the paper in support of or opposed to the issue? Who is on the editorial board? Which member of the advocacy group is the most appropriate person to develop a relationship with the editorial board?

Next, a letter should be written to the editorial board stating the nature of the issue and requesting a meeting. A phone call to schedule the meeting should follow. Once scheduled, a team of two or three individuals from the advocacy group should develop a short presentation. It is helpful if one member of the team has expertise on the issue area and is viewed by the editorial board as a credible source. Prior to the meeting, it is important to confirm how much time is allotted for the presentation, including time needed for questions.

The presentation to the board should be practiced thoroughly with all presenters clearly understanding the goal of the meeting, the main points of the presentation, and what is being requested from the editorial board. Additional information, in the form of fact sheets and background material, should be available upon request. The editorial board should always be thanked for providing an opportunity to meet. It should *never* be assumed that anything said in an editorial board meeting is off-the-record.

Other Print Media

Other print media outlets include locally published magazines and newsletters. Each publication will have a policy for publishing letters and point-of-view articles. It is important to identify the primary target audiences for each publication. For example, some communities have a local business magazine, which is a good vehicle for reaching employers regarding issues that affect their employees or business practices. Submitting an article on the importance of smoke-free worksites or granting release time for wellness activities as an incentive to encourage employee fitness, will reach a target audience that can influence or institute policy change.

Many civic groups, volunteer organizations, neighborhood associations, and schools distribute newsletters to their members or parents. The local library may have a listing of community volunteer organizations that includes descriptions of the organizations, contact persons, and mailing addresses. Local organizations can be contacted to determine if they publish a newsletter, accept articles from nonmembers, and are interested in receiving articles on health-related issues for possible inclusion in their publications. Creating a data base of organizations that are responsive to receiving and publishing articles eases the task of regularly sending materials to a large audience.

Electronic Media

Electronic media outlets include radio, television, and electronic mail (e-mail). While only one newspaper may exist in the community, there may be a number of different radio stations to which people listen on their daily commutes, at work, or at home. Radio news programs and talk radio shows offer excellent opportunities for media advocacy.

Most *radio* stations have local news segments and welcome local public reactions to national, state, and local news. Cultivating relationships with news directors and becoming established as a reliable source of information on health-related issues provides opportunities (e.g., interviews) to put a policy spin on an issue. As interviews are usually short in duration (30 seconds or less), it is important to have a number of planned, concise points prepared.

Talk radio provides a much longer opportunity for sharing a message. Instead of a 30-second sound bite, talk radio allows time to discuss issues at length while reaching a specific, and often large, audience. As with any media outlet, it is important to become familiar with the show's format and target audience. Listening to the talk radio show will provide an awareness of the style of the show and its host (e.g., Does the host pit guests against each other to stir up controversy?). The market share and target audiences associated with particular programming can be obtained from the radio station. If the audience is the same as that being targeted through the advocacy campaign, the host or station manager is more likely to have an interest in airing the issue.

Public service announcements (PSAs) are used by licensed radio and television stations to meet the requirement of federal law to serve in the public interest. While there are production costs involved, PSAs can provide free air time to groups for which paid advertising would be cost prohibitive. For instance, the U.S. Office on Smoking and Health receives approximately $2 million per year in free air time for PSAs.[4]

In contrast, drawbacks to using PSAs include the following: (1) Competition for free air time can be fierce in local communities; (2) production costs can be expensive; (3) the sponsor of the PSA has no impact on the placement, penetration, or frequency once a PSA is submitted; (4) PSAs cannot be used to respond quickly to a public issue; and (5) there is no guarantee that the message will reach the desired target audience.[4]

Television offers similar opportunities to radio in the form of local news segments and talk shows. Local television stations often have news programs that cover human interest or health stories. The Public Affairs Director of the local station can assist in determining what local opportunities exist (e.g., a two-minute segment on the news at noon, 15 minutes on a Sunday morning broadcast). Cultivating a relationship with the reporter that covers health or political issues allows for increased likelihood of supportive television coverage.

As with talk radio interviews, it is important to become aware of the format and target audience of the television show. Watching local shows will help in determining the style of the host. The market share of the show and audience demographics (age, gender, race, socioeconomic status) can be obtained from the television station. Information about the show that should be determined prior to agreeing to an interview includes (1) what other guests will be on the program, (2) the length of the segment, (3) whether calls will be taken from viewers, and (4) whether the show will be live or taped. When being interviewed, it is important to wear dark clothes with conservative tailoring, breathe deeply and calmly, maintain a composed demeanor and voice, and respond with brief, clear, and concise answers.[5]

E-mail, a fairly new form of electronic media, provides access to local, state, national, and global information resources. E-mail can be used to send a letter to the editor of a local, state, or national newspaper, which allows immediate response to a public policy issue. All elected federal officials and many elected state officials have e-mail addresses. Available e-mail addresses can be found by searching government sites on the Internet.

Paid Media

The approaches presented thus far focus on media outlets that are free of cost. Advocacy campaigns that are supported by large budgets should consider placing paid advertisements in local newspapers, on radio and television, and on billboards. The use of paid media to influence policy change has many advantages over free media. With paid media, the customer maintains control over the content and timing of the message.[6]

Paid media can be used to (1) piggyback on current events (e.g., focus on a seemingly unrelated story and tie it to a public health issue); (2) compare, contrast, and put an event into context (e.g., "Each year tobacco kills more people than does AIDS, cocaine, heroin, alcohol, fires, car crashes, homicide, and suicide combined"); (3) respond quickly; (4) counter opposing advertising; (5) lend credibility; (6) react and respond (silence may be viewed as agreeing with an opposing position); (7) stir up controversy (e.g., the *Dangerous Promises* campaign billboards previously presented); (8) refocus attention on an issue; and (9) express appreciation to supporters.[6]

An example of using paid media can be illustrated by an advertisement, created and aired by the Center for Science in the Public Interest, that focused on McDonald's practice of using saturated fats to prepare fast foods. The advertisement was addressed to the Chairperson of the Board of McDonald's and indicated that McDonald's fried foods were prepared using beef tallow, which is very high in saturated fat, and suggested substituting it with vegetable oil. In this paid advertisement, the Center was able to inform the general public of the high saturated fat content of fried foods at fast food restaurants, appeal to the good sense of the chairperson of a major fast food chain, and suggest a policy change that would impact the health of millions of consumers.[6]

Some national organizations and government agencies (e.g., CDC) have copy-ready advertisements available for organizations to use. For example, the National Center for Tobacco-Free Kids has developed a number of advertisements that are suitable for newspapers, newsletters, and other publications. These particular advertisements focus on the tobacco companies practice of marketing to youth, campaign contributions by the tobacco industry to candidates running for elected office, and support for the FDA regulations regarding tobacco sales to minors.

Framing the Issue

Framing the issue is the process of identifying how the issue will be depicted; it is "the package in which the main point of the story is developed, supported, and understood."[2] The impact of an issue on an individual's life is often of more interest to news reporters than the policy implications of an issue. Readers and viewers are more likely to identify emotionally with a person's plight.

It is important to frame the issue for both *access* and *content*. Framing the issue for *access* involves gaining access to the media by making the issue newsworthy. It provides visibility, credibility, and legitimacy for the issue so that media will have interest in covering it.[2] The following questions can help determine newsworthiness:

- Is the issue controversial (e.g., freedom of speech versus encouraging the sale of illegal products to minors)?

- Is there a milestone event (e.g., the introduction of FDA regulations)?

- Is there an anniversary (e.g., release of the Surgeon General's report on health consequences of tobacco use)?

- Can irony be used (e.g., after decades of denial, one tobacco company admits that smoking is addictive)?

- Can celebrities be used (e.g., local sports star comes out against spit tobacco use)?

- Does the issue connect with a larger, national event (e.g., local night spots go smoke-free for the *Great American Smoke Out*)?

Framing the issue for *content* shifts the individual problem to a social issue. For example, there is a current trend in many state legislatures to introduce youth tobacco access laws that heavily penalize youth who are attempting to purchase tobacco and clerks who sell tobacco products, but not the store owners. A way to frame this issue for content is to focus on the fact that tobacco companies market tobacco products to youth using images that are appealing to this age group, such as cartoon characters, men who are ruggedly independent and rebellious, and thin, independent females. The primary responsibility for the social issue of youth sales is shifted from individuals to tobacco industry marketing tactics.

INCREASING LIKELIHOOD OF SUCCESS

Regardless of how well formulated, even the best plans leave room for error. Consideration of the following activities may improve the likelihood of media advocacy success.

Recruiting Volunteers

One person cannot be expected to complete all the activities necessary for a well-rounded media advocacy campaign. Volunteers with an interest and stake in the issue are critical for success. A local coalition that addresses and focuses on impacting the issue of concern is the most logical place to recruit volunteers. If a local coalition does not exist, a state or national organization may already be working on the issue. For example, Mothers Against Drunk Driving (MADD) focuses on drinking and driving issues; the American Cancer Society, American Lung Association, and American Heart Association target tobacco issues; and Parents as Resources in Drug Education (PRIDE) focuses on alcohol and other drug issues. Youth-oriented national groups also exist, such as Students Against Drunk Driving (SADD) and the Smoke-Free Class of 2000. Local organizations (e.g., the United Way) and voluntary agencies (e.g., American Cancer Society, American Lung Association, and American Heart Association) can assist in identifying other groups that are working on similar issues. These organizations may also be able to provide a connection to state and national groups.

Local health departments and other health care providers can also be a source for volunteers.

Advertising for volunteers can occur through a number of professional and personal networking avenues (e.g., school PTAs, worksites, church groups). In addition, a simple survey can be developed and filled out by individuals attending advocacy meetings, health fairs, or other health promotion activities (see Figure 8-3). Advertising media advocacy as part of a presentation or display may also attract volunteers.

The number of people needed to run an effective media advocacy campaign depends on the scope of the campaign and the policy issue

Figure 8-3. Media Advocacy Survey

Name: _____

Organization: _____

Address: _____

_____

Phone Number: _____   Fax Number: _____

I am willing to write a Letter to the Editor about the following issues (check all that apply):

__ Tobacco   __ Environmental Health   __ Parenting   __ Cancer

__ Heart Health __ Infant Mortality   __ AIDS   __ Other

I am willing to serve as a media spokesperson about the following areas (check all that apply):

__ Tobacco   __ Environmental Health   __ Parenting   __ Cancer

__ Heart Health __ Infant Mortality   __ AIDS   __ Other

I know and am willing to talk with the following media people about health-related issues:

Name   Media Outlet (i.e., newspaper, radio, t.v.)

_____   _____

_____   _____

_____   _____

I am willing to help, but would like some training first in the following areas (check all that apply):

__ How to write a letter to the editor   __ How to be interviewed on radio

__ How to be a media spokesperson   __ How to be interviewed on television

__ Other: _____

being addressed. Having four to six individuals willing to write letters to the editor and serve as spokespersons on an issue is a good place to start. It is important to continually recruit and train volunteers to be media advocates in order to counter volunteer turnover and burn out.

Developing a Media Contact List

A list of local media contacts should be compiled. Each entry on the list should include (1) the name of the reporter; (2) telephone and fax numbers; (3) e-mail and mailing addresses; (4) the name of the newspaper, magazine, or station; (5) the best time to be reached; (6) sections or segments in which the reporter writes or reports (e.g., sports, columnist, lifestyle, health); and (7) a list of requirements for news avenues (e.g., press releases, announcements, community events listings). This should be updated regularly due to the high rate of turnover in the media.

Localizing the Issue

State or national data that relate to the advocacy issue should be localized whenever possible. Inversely, local data that relate to state or national issues should be utilized if available. Also, an individual in the community who has been affected by the issue could be solicited to either talk with the media or submit a letter to the editor. It is important to gain permission before sharing the individual's name and telephone number with a member of the media.

Timing Stories and Releases

Letters and other forms of releases (e.g., press releases, PSAs) need to be timely. A general rule of thumb is the sooner the better, but not more than four weeks ahead of the event. Local media contacts should be able to provide insight on timing. Once an article has been submitted, a follow-up should occur if further detail or information is needed.

Reviewing Local Periodicals

All sections of the local newspaper should be regularly scanned for articles that directly or indirectly relate to the advocacy issue. For instance, the sports page may cover an automobile race that is tobacco sponsored. This would be applicable for an advocacy campaign that focuses on supporting policy to ban tobacco sponsored sporting events. Articles that relate to the advocacy issue should be clipped and responded to by way of an op-ed or letter to the editor. Copies of the article can be sent to other community activists and appropriate legislators.

Providing Spokesperson Training

Members and volunteers associated with the advocacy campaign should receive training on effective use of media and interviewing skills. A training that allows practice on answering questions and sticking to the purpose of the interview will reduce nervousness and incidences of providing faulty information. Local media personalities may help locate a media specialist to assist in the training.

STRATEGIES FOR OVERCOMING BARRIERS

A number of potential barriers may threaten the success of the media advocacy campaign:

- Media advocacy can be a full-time job and is, usually, added on to a full schedule or work load.

- By nature, media advocacy is controversial. Communities are asked to examine their values, making it difficult to convince individuals to get involved.

- Those who are successful media advocates find that the opposition responds by increasing money, resources, and counter messages aimed at defeating the advocacy message.

- Reporters may call for information when the media advocate has not had time to prepare a statement on an issue.

- With the enormity of individual public health issues, it may be challenging to decide where to focus and what impact is realistic.

In order to effectively accomplish advocacy goals, the above mentioned problems need to be planned for accordingly. One way to reduce the impact of potential barriers is to start small and keep it simple. A letter to the editor, which is read by many decision makers and opinion leaders in the community, is a simple media advocacy activity. Being prepared further aids in deferring barriers. It is important to keep current with trends within a certain health-related area, and to collect and maintain statistics, fact sheets, and articles. Having a good library of materials on hand will help when an unexpected phone call comes from a media contact needing a comment on a newsworthy issue. Lists of media bites (i.e., short, factual, responses) should be prepared on a number of different topics. If a comment or statistic is not readily available, it is acceptable to ask for time to get back to the reporter. It is important to respond in a timely manner.

Any appearance on a television show or talk radio show should be rehearsed. Having a list of the key points about the issue will help in bringing the interviewer back to focus if the interview begins to digress. This list will also assist in preventing involvement in a debate or side issue. The following author experience illustrates this process:

> *Once when I was interviewed about the proposed FDA regulations regarding access of youth to tobacco products, the reporter asked what I thought about the fact that the President Clinton smoked cigars. I replied that the President was of legal age to smoke cigars and though I would not recommend it, the important focus was on the ground breaking proposal to keep tobacco products out of the hands of minors.*

Advocacy success can also be increased by taking advantage of training opportunities that exist for public speaking, writing for the media, and media advocacy. The Advocacy Institute is an excellent resource for media advocacy. The Benton Foundation has a publication series, *Strategic Communications for Nonprofits,* which includes booklets on media advocacy and op-eds. Many other organizations have materials and strategies for media advocacy or presentations (see Table 8-1).

EXPECTED OUTCOMES

A well-planned media advocacy campaign can be expected to, at the least, increase media coverage of an issue. Over time, a shift in attitudes or be-

Table 8-1. Resources for Media Advocacy

The Advocacy Institute
1707 L Street NW, Suite 400
Washington, DC 20036
(202) 659-8475

Benton Foundation
134 Eye Street, NW, 12th floor
Washington, DC 20006
(202) 638-5770
benton@benton.org
http://www.benton.org

National Center for Tobacco-Free Kids
1707 L Street NW, Suite 800
Washington, DC 20036
(202) 296-5469

haviors by the general public or target audiences should occur. The optimal outcome of media advocacy is policy change. Due to media advocacy being one of many strategies used to promote policy change, however, it may be difficult to isolate its precise contribution to a successful (or unsuccessful) policy initiative.[2]

In determining success, both the *process* and *impact* of the campaign should be considered. Three questions can be used to serve as a guide for evaluating the *process* of the media advocacy campaign: (1) Was the issue covered by the media? (2) was the issue framed with a policy spin? and (3) was the issue pushed forward by the media focus? Avenues for determining the extent of the process could include identifying the amount and placement of media coverage, conducting a content analysis (e.g., did the stories focus on broad policy issues or on individual victims and their situations?), and keeping track of the progress of the desired policy change.[2]

Questions that focus on evaluating the *impact* of the campaign include the following: (1) Did the issue reach the attention of the public? (2) were policy makers or decision makers influenced to support the policy change? and (3) was the policy adopted or did change occur? Strategies and approaches should be reviewed over time, especially because policy changes can take years to enact.[2]

Does media advocacy work? Qualitative evidence from a number of campaigns designed to address health problems including alcohol, tobacco, HIV/AIDS, and gun violence indicates that media advocacy should be considered by health educators as an effective mechanism for enacting change.[2] The *Dangerous Promises* campaign previously presented is a prime example of effective media advocacy influencing policy change.

A recent issue of *The Cancer Letter* reported that the media advocacy aspect of the American Stop Smoking Intervention Study (ASSIST) demonstration program had been successful.[7] As part of the National Cancer Institute's three- to four-year evaluation of the ASSIST project, the following results were found:

> *State legislatures, local governments, or major institutions in all 17 states have introduced or strengthened tobacco control and clean indoor air regulations, including increasing taxes on tobacco products and instituting smoking bans in public places and workplace smoking policies. . . . Newspapers in ASSIST states have published 25 percent more stories about tobacco than have papers in non-ASSIST states. Of these stories, 85 percent had a point of view that was either neutral or in favor of tobacco control. . . . More than 30 shopping malls in 10 ASSIST states have adopted smoke-free policies.*

CONCLUSION

Many of the examples in this chapter focused on tobacco because tobacco issues currently dominate many health-related media advocacy efforts. Media advocacy, however, can be used to change public opinion and policies in any health-related area. Once the policy goal has been set, a media advocacy campaign can be developed by following five basic steps: (1) Know who needs to be reached, (2) decide what is to be accomplished, (3) determine what resources and information are needed, (4) find out how to access the media, and (5) decide how to frame the issue. Media advocacy can be controversial, which is good because policy change and shifts in public opinion often begin with controversy. Properly implemented, it can create lasting change toward healthier communities.

References

1. Woodruff, K. (1996). Alcohol advertising and violence against women: A media advocacy case study. *Health Education Quarterly, 23,* 330-345.

2. Wallack, L., & Dorfman, L. (1996). Media advocacy: A strategy for advancing policy and promoting health. *Health Education Quarterly, 23,* 293-317.

3. Zeck, D., & Rennolds, E. (1991). *Op-Eds.* Washington, D.C.: Benton Foundation.

4. Pertschuk, M., & Wilbur, P. (1991). Reframing public debate. In L. Kirkman & K. Menichelli (Eds.), *Media advocacy.* Washington, D.C.: Benton Foundation.

5. Mallory, C. (1989). *Publicity power: A practical guide to effective promotion.* Los Altos, CA: Crisp Publications.

6. O'Keefe, A. (1991). A case for paid media. In L. Kirkman & K. Menichelli (Eds.), *Media advocacy.* Washington, D.C.: Benton Foundation.

7. Goldberg, K. B., & Goldberg, P. (Eds.). (1997). ASSIST gets extra year of funding while NCI considers role in tobacco control. *The Cancer Letter, 23*(2), 1-5.

Chapter 9

LEGISLATIVE INVOLVEMENT AND ACTION

Michelle Baukema, B.A.A.

Author's Comments: *For most of the seven years that I have spent in health education, I have been working on tobacco reduction related activities. Looking back, it feels like much of this time was dedicated to legislative work. You see, the legislative engines never stop working. Upon completion of one task, you are immediately faced with another. That is what makes legislative advocacy so exciting. Change is continuous, especially if your topic is hot enough, like tobacco or sex education. Even more important than the public view of the topic is the commitment and energy you give to it. Spirit catches on. If you are excited and can show people how to get involved, you are that much further along.*

I have found that individual members of groups that are aware of the need for and have acquired skills associated with legislative involvement are more than willing to write or call their legislators. The first time, however, can be a frightening experience. The first time I called the Governor's office to discuss preemption of local tobacco reduction laws, I was so nervous that I could barely provide my name and explain the reason for the call. After the first few minutes, however, I rolled right into my points and had a somewhat pleasant conversation with the Governor's aide. Contrary to public opinion, legislators do listen. It is their job, even if they have to be reminded of it once in a while.

Mastery of legislative advocacy comes with experience. But even then, something new can always be learned. Give yourself time to experience the process and try different ways of communicating with your legislator. You will find that what works is totally dependent on the legislator. As you will find in this chapter, and in other readings on legislative advocacy, there are no absolutes. The intent of this chapter is to provide ground level education, suggestions on how to start, and how the legislative process works.

INTRODUCTION

Health educators are involved in the legislative process in many ways, because so much of what they do is dictated by legislative policy. For instance, much of the funding for HIV/AIDS prevention and treatment in the U.S. comes from federal legislation. Health educators must be involved with and constantly monitoring the policies that govern these funds. If legislation changed, many health education services would cease to exist.

Health educators have also joined the legislative arena because large amounts of funding for salaries are dictated by legislation. This occurs directly by law, or through state or federal agencies that depend on legislation to support their budgets. For instance, many tobacco reduction efforts across the U.S. are being funded from the National Cancer Institute, which receives funding from the federal government. Again, involvement and monitoring is required to ensure that funding continues to be provided.

Without the legislative involvement of health educators, programs can easily be lost in the political shuffle. Health educators may find themselves involved in the legislative process by providing testimony at a hearing, writing or calling elected officials, finding community members to support a bill or existing policy, or advocating with local government officials to change laws. For these reasons, legislative involvement and action should be an integral part of every health agency. Health educators should also know that when it comes to legislative advocacy, nothing is more effective than a well-educated, unified voice.

This chapter will provide practitioners with practical steps to involvement in the legislative process, tips and techniques for successful legislative campaigns, strategies for overcoming barriers, and expected outcomes of political involvement. Throughout the chapter, the terms "legislator," "policy maker," and "official" will be used interchangeably. Other terms common to legislative issues, are listed in Table 9-1.[1-3]

STEPS TO LEGISLATIVE INVOLVEMENT AND ACTION

Health educators must understand the process of legislative involvement and action prior to becoming involved. Four crucial steps to legislative involvement include (1) identifying policy makers, (2) selecting a legislative issue, (3) establishing grass roots movements for legislative action, and (4) introducing and tracking a legislative issue.

Identifying Policy Makers

A list of local policy makers can be obtained from any city, township, or county office. Also available are the office addresses and telephone numbers, office hours, and committee assignments (e.g., budget and finance, health policy, transportation) of each elected official. In some states, these are readily available as policy makers are continually improving ways to be more accessible to their constituency. For instance, some officials offer

Table 9-1: Legislative Terms

Advocacy: A catchall phrase for the set of skills used to create a shift in public opinion, money, and other resources, to support an issue, policy or constituency.

Campaign: A set of actions, with specified objectives and time lines, undertaken to effect policy change.

Community Influentials: Persons living in a particular district or city with common interests, work, etc., who have the ability or power to affect others either directly or indirectly (e.g., through influence, authority, prestige, reputation).

Law: A principle governing action or procedure.

Legislator: A citizen who is elected to represent the people either on the local, state, or federal level for the purpose of enacting laws. Also called policy maker, commissioner, township supervisor, etc.

Lobbying: To support a certain piece of legislation.

Lobbyist: A person who works to promote the passage of legislation by influencing public officials.

Policy Maker: Anyone who makes policy, such as Rotary committees, college administrators, and PTA members. Every institution makes policy. Therefore, every institution has policy makers.

Policy Initiative: An action or set of actions undertaken to change policy or put pressure on a institution to enforce existing policies.

"coffee hours" at local establishments in their districts. This allows constituents to meet with their policy makers without an appointment. Others may travel around their districts, and speak or meet with constituents. Knowing the civic groups of which the official is a member (e.g., Lions Club, Rotary Club) provides insight into personal interests and community commitment, and will help in determining allies or opponents for legislative concerns.

A legislative directory from elected officials' offices can assist in determining state and federal officials. For instance, many state legislators in Michigan provide the booklet *A Citizen's Guide to State Government* free to constituents. Within the guide are state and federal legislators' mailing addresses, telephone and fax numbers, and committee assignments. The guide also lists the addresses for state and federal executive branches. In addition to this type of directory, many legislators can be reached through the Internet via state or federal legislative home pages.

It is also important to know when policy makers' committees and board meetings occur. Any official's office staff can assist with this information. At the local level, newspapers usually print committee and board meeting information a week in advance. In order to become familiar with the meeting style of the board or committee, as well as to meet committee members, a health educator should attend a few meetings before introducing a legislative issue to the group.

State legislators usually split time between the Capital and their individual districts. In Michigan, for example, legislators are typically in respective districts on Monday and Friday, while the rest of week is spent at the Capital working on legislative issues. It is usually easier to speak with legislators when they are in their local districts. If at the Capital, however, an opportunity to meet legislators and their staff should never be missed. Even though it is better to schedule an appointment to meet with a legislator, it is acceptable to stop by an official's office without an appointment. If the official is not available, the health educator should request to speak with a staff member and, if predetermined, leave material about the legislative issue.

Selecting a Legislative Issue

After identifying the policy makers, the next step is choosing a legislative or policy issue to support, or in some cases, oppose. There are basically three types of policies, which are presented in the following according to their level of difficulty.

Voluntary policies, which are the most basic type of policy issues, are issues that individual institutions (e.g., worksites, community settings), or persons, choose to implement without government direction. For example, a magazine can enact a policy to not advertise alcohol or tobacco products in their publication. This action is done based on the magazine's principles, versus being required by law. *Local ordinances* are enacted by government bodies to change policy at the local level (e.g., city, township, or county). For example, a county board of commissioners may mandate smoke-free buildings in private worksites for businesses registered within the county. *State and federal laws* are enacted by legislators to change policy at the state and federal levels. For instance, a state may enact specific penalties for drunk driving in its state. State and federal laws are more difficult policies for health educators to influence.

For many community coalitions and groups, the process of selecting a policy issue is one that is determined by the group's prior experiences with advocacy. As the group matures, advocacy efforts should move from easy to more difficult types of policy issues. If a group has never engaged in an advocacy effort, they would be better served by choosing an issue which is less difficult. This would enable the members to learn how to work together and develop advocacy strategies. The process could be started by encouraging the adoption of a voluntary policy, such as encouraging restaurants to go smoke-free on their own, instead of pursing a city ordinance to ban smoking in restaurants. The latter requires more experience and planning on the group's behalf, while the former can sometimes be achieved by just changing one person's mind (i.e., the restaurant owner).

Success with a basic policy issue will build strength, increase team spirit, and expand membership of the group for future endeavors. Success breeds success. As other community members see the success and determination of the group, more advocates will likely be attracted, thus allowing the group to choose more challenging legislative issues.

Before choosing an issue, however, the group (e.g., coalition) or organization will want to evaluate its assets and liabilities to ensure resources needed for committing to a campaign are in place. This planning will help avoid pitfalls once the campaign begins. For example, when community support for a policy does not exist, it is important for the group to enact strategies to gain support prior to contacting policy makers. Having resources such as constituent support for an issue, improves the likelihood that the policy maker will be interested in the group's position. Examples of constituent support include letters of support, letters to the editor, public demonstrations, and telephone calls to legislators supporting the proposed law. In order to evaluate resources needed for success, a number of questions should be considered before pursuing a legislative issue:[2]

- What will be gained or lost by supporting or opposing the issue?

- What is the experience and commitment of the membership?

- Is there sufficient staff for a legislative campaign?

- What funding is available to support the campaign? (Some funding agencies and grant funds have specific guidelines about legislative involvement. This should be determined beforehand in case alternative funding is needed.)

- What community resources (e.g., money, space, materials) are available?

- Who are the group's allies and adversaries on this issue?

- Who else shares this problem (groups or individuals)?

- What would those groups who share the problem gain or lose by joining the campaign?

- What laws, if any, already exist to deal with the issue of concern?

Finally, the group must determine what rules and regulations exist that govern their involvement in legislative advocacy. The group does not want to lose momentum because they did not follow guidelines established by the organizational leadership. For instance, many health educators work in public health settings (e.g., health departments, hospitals), and as part of their job responsibilities, lead community groups. In this situation, they would be well advised to check with leaders of their organization (e.g., health officer, hospital administrator) before committing to an advocacy campaign. By thoroughly investigating the issue and knowing all of the angles beforehand, the health educator can avoid many mistakes and be better prepared for challenges.

Establishing Grass Roots Movements for Legislative Action

Grass roots movements are typically known as alliances of local people voluntarily working together toward a common goal. People usually feel more confident and willing to tackle legislative issues when they are part of a group in which members have similar beliefs. Forming a group to advocate for or against an issue is often more effective than an individual voice because a group can share responsibilities and complete more tasks. For example, when groups like the American Cancer Society, American Lung Association, and American Heart Association join forces in Washington, DC, they are representing hundreds of thousands of individual voices. Policy makers listen because they know that some of their constituents are a part of these groups. A grass roots group can formulate for either a short- or long-term legislative initiative. The following are suggestions for organizing grass roots efforts for a legislative campaign.

Forming a Steering Committee
Even though a grass roots effort can be loosely organized, it still requires a leader, and a handful of individuals, to share in the decision-making process. Recruiting community influentials, organizations, and community members who have the ability to affect change, are good choices for membership on a steering committee. These individuals usually have the skills and resources (e.g., experience, political connections) to help make the campaign a success. The health educator's role in forming a steering committee could be to bring concerned parties together and facilitate meetings.

Selecting a Chairperson
The chairperson of the group should be a community member who possesses skills associated with leadership, negotiation, communication, delegation, and meeting management. Choosing a person with these skills will allow the group to efficiently move though the planning process and on to the challenge of policy advocacy. The chairperson will also serve as liaison to the community and media.

Setting Goals and Priorities
Once a chair is selected, the group should set goals and prioritize tasks for the campaign. Such tasks include developing a goal statement, handling

media, recruiting members, developing a budget, developing an information campaign, and polling policy makers. Setting goals and priorities will
provide organization and a systematic approach to the legislative issue.
These priorities can be either sequentially or simultaneously addressed.
For instance, polling officials to determine support for the policy or ordinance, and contacting government offices for procedure in introducing
policy issues, could be done at the same time.

Assigning Tasks

Once priorities are set, small groups, or subcommittees, will be most effective at achieving the goals, because all members can participate within their
levels of expertise and time allowances. For instance, someone who has
difficulty coming to meetings can be asked to stuff envelopes for a mailing.
During group meetings, ample time should be allowed for subcommittees
to report on progress and troubleshoot problem areas.

Educating Community Members and Policy Makers

Any legislative initiative will require developing an information campaign.
This achieves two purposes: (1) To educate the community and policy
makers about the issue, and (2) to move the public into action. Several
strategies that can be used in an information campaign are listed in Table
9-2. It is important to make sure the information being shared is accurate
and provided in an easy-to-understand way.

Introducing a Legislative Issue

Local policy issues are fairly easy to introduce. By contacting the local governing body in which the policy is to be introduced, the group will be able
to determine the best approach. The group should also choose a spokes-

Table 9-2. Information Campaign Strategies

- Writing letters to the editor.
- Meeting with the local newspaper editorial board to discuss writing an article in favor of the issue.
- Paying for advertisements, if the budget allows.
- Developing pamphlets and flyers that describe the issue and give a task to the reader (e.g., write or call an official, join the group, tell a friend, participate in a protest).
- Holding forums for the public and policy makers to share information.
- Utilizing group members' personal and professional contacts to find additional opportunities to present the issue.
- Tracking legislation and testifying at hearings.

person for this task. Each group member's previous experience with the legislative committee (positive or negative), reputation in the community, personal or professional experience with the issue, and association with the group, should be considered. For example, in introducing a policy on maintenance and safety checks for park equipment, a parent of a child who was injured on a poorly maintained playground may be an excellent choice as a spokesperson on this issue. Table 9-3 provides the process that is normally followed once a local (in this example, county) policy issue has been introduced.[1]

At the state and federal level, the policy issue must be introduced to the legislature. This occurs either in the House of Representatives, the Senate, or both simultaneously. A member of the group or the group's lobbyist needs to bring the issue to a legislator (preferably one who supports the issue), who can then introduce the issue into the legislature.

Once introduced, the issue will be processed as a bill. If passed by both the House and Senate, the bill becomes a law. Table 9-4 outlines the steps of how a bill becomes a law.[4]

Evaluating Progress

Periodic review of the campaign's progress will determine (1) if objectives are being met, (2) if members feel satisfied with involvement, (3) what barriers continue to exist, and (4) the future direction of the initiative. Evaluation can occur in many ways. For example, members could be polled as to their achievements and challenges, or a list of where policy makers stand on the issue could be tallied and shared with members. Assessing what has been changed (e.g., policy, community opinion, policy maker's stance), what still needs to be done, and what is not working, all provide important information in determining the success or failure of the campaign.

TIPS AND TECHNIQUES FOR SUCCESS

All too often, legislation is enacted, changed, or dissolved without the public's knowledge. Elected officials need to know how their constituents feel about the issues. If policy makers do not hear from their constituency, their may vote on issues may not reflect the opinions of the community, which could result in the passing of a law that will hurt, more than help, the people of their district. Therefore, legislative initiatives will always be enhanced through personal involvement. Campaigns take planning and creativity to spark community participation. Providing useful ways for the public to get involved will help further the campaign. Strategies for getting the public involved include (1) legislative alerts, (2) letter writing campaigns, (3) personal contacts with legislators, (4) testifying at hearings, and (5) media advocacy.

Legislative Alerts

Legislative alerts are notices to group members about upcoming votes, needed action (e.g., letter or phone call to official), committee meetings, or hearings. A successful alert will contain a summary of the issue, the position of the group, background information, and the action needed by the individual or group receiving the information. To make contacting a policy maker easier, the official's name, address, and phone number, should be strategically placed on the alert. Development of a fax and phone tree beforehand will cut down on time spent placing calls. A simple message, accompanied by a specific action, will help ensure the alert is understood.

Letter Writing Campaigns

Letter writing campaigns are used to educate and urge policy makers to act. A successful campaign will encompass the same qualities as a legisla-

Table 9-3. Steps for Passing a County Regulation

1.	Coalition raises an issue to the health department of the county government.
2.	Health officer or other community leader introduces idea to the Board of Health.
3.	Regulation language (how the bill will be written) is researched (e.g., examples from other areas that already have a similar law are collected).
4.	Language is drafted and reviewed by the County Attorney.
5.	Regulation language and data are presented to the Board of Health.
6.	The Board of Health holds meetings or hearings to discuss the proposed regulation.
7.	Once passed by the Board of Health, the regulation is presented to the County Board of Commissioners for approval.
8.	A task force may be appointed to research the regulation, table it, or refer it to another committee for their recommendation.
9.	Public hearing dates are set (normally three dates).
10.	Notification of dates are announced in the local newspaper.
11.	Public hearing(s) are held in which the community has the opportunity to present arguments for or against the proposed regulation.
12.	Commissioners vote on the regulation.
13.	If passed by the Board of Commissioners, the local health department has authority to adopt the regulation.

Note: This process may vary depending on locality and individual issues.

tive alert, but with more detail. A campaign can begin before or after an issue is introduced in a legislative body. To help in letter writing, a sample letter for members to sign, and personalize with their thoughts, should be used. Often, response to letter writing campaigns is small because people are unaware of what to do. Names should be spelled out and the letter proofread prior to sending. Letters from constituents that are handwritten, individually authored, or neatly typed are better received by legislators than form letters. A handwritten letter shows that time and thoughtfulness on the part of the author went into the letter. When time is of the essence, however, a signed form letter is better than no correspondence at all. The following writing tips will increase the likelihood of writing an impacting letter.[4]

- *Address the letter properly.* Use the legislator's full name:

  For a U.S. Senator: *For a State Representative:*

  The Honorable (full name)   The Honorable (full name)
  United States Senator   State Representative
  State Capital   State Capital
  Address   Address

  Dear Senator (last name):   Dear Representative (last name):

- *Always include your name and address on the letter.* A letter cannot be answered if no return address exists, or the signature is not legible.

- *Use your own words.* In general, legislators do not like form letters. These are identified as organized pressure campaigns, and are often answered with form replies. As stated previously, however, sending sample letters to members helps organize thoughts. If time is of the essence, a form is better than no letter.

- *Timing is everything.* Write the legislator and the chair of the committee in which the bill is assigned while the bill is still in committee. This will allow for optimal impact. If this cannot be done, send the letter anyway, as it still alerts the policy maker of the concern.

- *Identify the bill by number or by title.* For instance, "House Bill 2440" is a bill number, while "Healthy Michigan Fund" is a bill title. The Secretary of the Senate or Clerk of the House will have information about the bill of interest. Call the state Capital and ask for these persons, or call the sponsoring legislator's office.

- *Be brief and constructive.* State the facts, the group's proposals, solutions, and personal positions on the matter. A one-page letter is greatly appreciated and welcomed by most legislators.

When disagreeing with a bill or policy, be constructive and offer solutions, or state a better way to approach the issue.

- *Request a response.* Responses are not always sent. Asking for one in your letter, however, will increase the likelihood of receiving a response. Follow-up with the legislator's office if a reply is not received.

- *Send a thank you.* If legislators have taken action that is appreciated, thank them. Legislating can be a thankless job, so recognizing a legislator's efforts is all the more important to maintaining good relations.

Personal Contact with Legislators

Contact from within the policy maker's constituency is crucial. Policy makers are elected by their local constituency to represent them in a larger arena (e.g., city, county, state, federal). What is most important about writing, calling, and meeting with legislators is that it reminds them that the issue is supported by the local constituents. It also makes the legislators keenly aware that someone is concerned and watching their actions. The following suggestions are useful when contacting legislators:[5]

- *Identify policy makers.* A card file listing elected officials should be created for each member. This will help when asking members to contact legislators.

- *Determine members that have personal contacts with policy makers.* Being on a first name basis improves access to officials, and personal and professional relationships with policy makers can be an advantage. Members who know officials may be able to get them to more readily listen to an issue.

- *Know the facts.* Before contacting the policy maker, all sides of the issue should be researched for a clear understanding of the facts about the issue. The policy maker's position on the issue should be found out ahead of time so the group can argue persuasively. Although expertise is not required, the group must appear well informed.

- *Know when and how to contact policy makers.* The group should be aware of when policy makers are at the Capital, versus their respective districts, prior to initiating a meeting. If the policy maker is unavailable, a meeting can be arranged with a legislative aide. Staff members are often more accessible, and will likely share your concerns with the official.

Table 9-4. How a Bill Becomes a Law

1. A bill is introduced in either the Senate or the House. Sometimes identical bills are simultaneously introduced. The bill receives FIRST READING (which means it is recognized as an issue and given a title and number) in the House and FIRST AND SECOND READING (which means it is reported back from committee and opportunity for full debate and amendment action occur) in the Senate (at which time the title is read). Then, the Majority Leader of the Senate or the Speaker of the House refers the bill to an appropriate standing committee (e.g., education, commerce, health). If the bill is a budget bill or has fiscal implications, it will be referred directly to the Appropriations Committee (a joint committee of the Senate and House), or to an appropriate standing committee and then to the Appropriations Committee.

2. In standing committee, the bill is discussed and debated. Public hearings may be held. Not every bill before the committee will be considered. The committee may take one of several different actions:
    *   Report the bill with favorable recommendation.
    *   Add amendments and report the bill with favorable recommendation.
    *   Replace the original bill with a substitute.
    *   Report the bill with adverse recommendation.
    *   Report the bill without recommendation.
    *   Report the bill with amendments but without recommendation.
    *   Report the bill with the recommendation that the bill be referred to another committee.
    *   Take no action on the bill.
    *   Refuse to report the bill out of committee.

3. If a bill is reported out favorably or a substitute is offered, the bill is returned to the Senate or House where it receives a GENERAL ORDERS status in the Senate and SECOND READING status in the House. The Senate resolves itself into the Committee-of-the-Whole (the entire Senate sitting as a committee and operating under informal rules) and the House assumes the order of SECOND READING. At this time, committee recommendations are considered and amendments may be offered and adopted. The bill then advances to THIRD READING (the final stage of consideration of a legislative bill before a vote on its final form).

4. Upon THIRD READING in the Senate, an entire bill is read unless unanimous consent is given to consider the bill read. In the House, the bill is read in its entirety on THIRD READING unless four-fifths of the members consent to consider the bill read. At THIRD READING the bill is again subject to debate and amendment. At the conclusion of THIRD READING, the bill is either passed or defeated by a roll call vote of the majority of members elected and serving, **OR** one of the following options may be used to delay final action:
    *   Refer bill back to committee for further consideration.
    *   Postpone bill indefinitely.
    *   Make the bill a special order of business on THIRD READING for a specific date.
    *   Table the bill.
    *   Following either passage or defeat of a bill, a legislator may move to have the bill reconsidered. In the Senate the motion must be made within the next two session days; in the House by the next day.

Figure 9-4 (continued).

5. If the bill passes, it goes to the other legislative branch (i.e., House or Senate) where the same procedure is followed. If the bill is passed in the same form by both houses, it is ordered "enrolled" in the house in which it originated. It then goes to the Governor (or President) for signature.

6. If the bill is passed in a different form by the second house, the bill is returned to its house of origin. If this house accepts the changes, the bill is enrolled and sent to the Governor (or President). If the changes are rejected, the bill is sent to a conference committee that tries to resolve differences. If the first conference report is rejected, a second conference committee may be appointed.

7. The Governor (or President) has 14 days after receiving a bill to consider it. The bill may be:
   • Signed. The bill becomes law either 90 days after the legislature adjourns at the end of the year or at a later date specified in the bill. If the bill has been given immediate effect by a two-thirds vote of the members elected and serving, it becomes law upon the Governor's (or President's) signature.
   • Vetoed (can be overridden by a two-thirds vote by both houses).
   • Neither signed nor vetoed, in which case the bill becomes law 14 days after reaching the Governor's desk, unless the legislature adjourns at the end of the year within the 14 days. In that case, the bill does not become law.

8. If the Governor (or President) vetoes a bill while the legislature is in session or recess, one of the following actions may occur:
   • The legislature may override the veto by a two-thirds vote of the members elected and serving in both houses.
   • Bill may not receive the necessary two-thirds vote and thus the attempt to override the veto will fail.
   • Bill may be tabled pending an attempt to override the veto.
   • Bill may be re-referred to a committee.

Note: In general, this process is the same throughout the Unites States. However, health educators should confer with their state's legislative processes.

• *Be an expert.* Expertise on an issue should be shared with a policy maker. Because policy makers cannot be experts on everything, many welcome expert knowledge.

• *Send members to talk with policy makers.* A crowd will not be necessary to get a message across. A few members that well-represent the group can be effective. A primary spokesperson (perhaps the group chairperson) should be selected to keep the meeting personal and substantive.

• *Keep it simple.* By selecting a few pertinent pieces of information about the issue, and presenting these to the policy maker during a face-to-face meeting, members will stay on task. A cover letter providing a brief overview of the group's position and a business card for follow-up should be left for the policy maker. Overkill with reports and handouts is not necessary.

- *Remain calm.* Even when the legislator disagrees with the group's position on an issue, members need to remain calm and polite. By listening to arguments and taking notes, facts will be generated. Understanding where the official is coming from may help in developing counter arguments.

- *Be patient.* Once information is presented, a few days should be given for the policy maker to review the issue. The bill or policy must be tracked as it moves through the legislative process. This is necessary because officials may need to be approached several times, from a number of different angles, before supporting the issue.

Testifying at a Hearing

The purpose of a committee hearing is to obtain written and oral testimony on a bill. Before the start of the hearing, audience members are usually able to submit testifying cards, which include the individual's name, organization, and position on the bill. Even if not testifying, a card indicating support or opposition to the bill should be completed, as all completed cards are filed and tabulated for the record. The following suggestions increase the likelihood of success in testifying.[4,6]

- *Prepare a written statement in advance.* Keep it brief. Usually, each person testifying is allotted 2-3 minutes. Comments should be practiced ahead of time by highlighting one or two points from the written statement. Before testifying, a person's name, organization, and position on the bill should be stated.

- *Use sound bites (catchy phrases).* The official will remember sound bites and the press will quote them. For example: "The number of tobacco-related deaths each year is equal to two jumbo jets crashing every day for a year."

- *Use personal experiences to enhance testimony.* For instance, personal insight on how drunk driving has affected families, or how barriers to health care has diminished a child's health may be helpful. Avoid overly emotional testimony and alienating committee members.

- *Listen to prior speakers.* By taking notes, those testifying can avoid repeating previously stated facts. When it is time to speak, offer highlights of the prepared testimony and ask that the full written testimony be placed in record for the committee to review at future meetings.

- *Observe the members of the committee.* Watch officials' body language, and comments to one another and other speakers. Change testimony if needed, or reinforce a previous point made with additional facts.

- *Expect questions or comments.* When answering a question, improvisation is not recommended. This is not the time for misinformation, especially if asked about a report or document that has never been seen. Ask for a copy of the document to review. By providing written comments later, misinformation will be avoided. If a hostile response is received from committee members, stay calm and cool. Stop and think about the appropriate answer before responding.

- *Testifying in opposition to a bill.* If a bill will be opposed, research the facts, consult with other professionals, and provide alternatives to the bill. Avoid complaining and stay focused on solving the problem.

Using Media for Legislative Advocacy

Effectively involving the media in a legislative campaign first requires establishing relationships with media personnel. This process can begin by getting to know the health writer for the newspaper, or the health reporter for the television station. The relationship should be cultivated before initiating the legislative campaign. Being on a first name basis with a reporter will help gain access and, hopefully, result in good media coverage of the campaign. Strategies for building media relationships include the following:[7]

- Involving members of the media in a training for group members on effectively communicating with the media. Bringing in members of media to the training accomplishes two goals: (1) The group can receive first hand strategies on how to utilize the media, and (2) it allows an opportunity for the media to be educated about the group's issues.

- Meeting with newspaper/magazine editors for advice on editorials.

- Researching and seeking alternatives from mainstream media. For instance, do culturally or racially specific media exist in the area?

- Participating in media sponsored community events that the group can support through personnel, promotion, or funding.

Establishing a media committee for the legislative campaign should be a consideration of the group. The committee objectives would be to increase public understanding of the issues, strengthen the public's desire to see changes made, and promote the larger group's goals. Utilizing the media in all forms can help reach the voting population in a fairly easy and timely fashion. Media can also be used to educate policy makers, members of the media, and the general public.

STRATEGIES FOR OVERCOMING BARRIERS

There are many barriers to legislative involvement; some being easier to overcome than others. The following are strategies for overcoming some of the more common barriers to legislative involvement and action.

Opposition Groups

It is important to be prepared for opposition to the issue. Become aware of opponents, their facts on the issue, and other groups' action plans. One strategy for accomplishing this task includes becoming a member of opposing groups. For example, in the tobacco arena, many tobacco-reduction advocates are on smokers' rights mailing lists in order to gather information. This tactic alerts the group to upcoming legislative initiatives that the opposition will be proposing, so appropriate strategies for combating them can be planned.

Lack of Community Support

Lack of community interest is a barrier most groups must deal with at one time or another. Just as there is attrition among group members of a committee, there will be attrition amongst the public towards the legislative advocacy effort. Even the largest, best facilitated groups struggle to keep the public aware of their issue. The group or organization should continually strive to provide clear, concise information with tasks for the member or community constituency to perform. Even basic citizenship rights must be reiterated, because too often people are unaware of their elected and appointed officials, and, therefore, are unsure of how to communicate with policy makers. The community should be educated about their representatives, and how the legislative process works, prior to asking them to perform a task for the legislative effort.

Volunteer Burnout

To combat volunteer burnout, short, time-specific opportunities for involvement should be provided to members. For example, two-hour shifts at a health fair provide members with opportunities to verbally share the organization's position and improve communication skills essential for future letter writing and testifying. People will often get involved once they are fully educated about the process, and have had task-specific opportunities for participation. Burnout will always occur, so new, fresh members should continually be recruited. For instance, authors of favorable letters to the editor can be contacted to join the group. Some local paper editors will relay messages to specific authors, if conventional ways of reaching them are unsuccessful.

Organizational Limitations

Limitations placed on the group regarding legislative activities may result due to the issue, players involved, funding, or agency rules and regulations. If limitations exist, then other ways of participating in the legislative process, without appearing like advocacy or lobbying efforts, should be determined. For instance, an organization could write a letter of support to a policy maker. The organization might also discuss the issue with supporters of the group who could, in turn, bring the issue to the policy maker's attention. Funding is typically a major limitation for groups in promoting their issues. As previously stated, a review of funding source stipulations about using funds toward legislative efforts should be conducted.

No Movement on a Policy

Bills and policies are often stalled in committee or never brought up for a hearing. Keeping track of the bill is the only way to monitor the process. When a bill is stalled, request that the chair of the committee be asked why the bill has not progressed, and that it be referred to another committee for consideration. Bills that have not been referred to another committee may have to be reintroduced to the committee during the next session. The bill can also be tacked onto another bill that has already passed the committee. The bill's sponsor should be contacted to determine the plausibility of this tact, as this procedure happens often and is a viable strategy for consideration.

EXPECTED OUTCOMES

It is often difficult to predict the outcome of legislative involvement and action, as many internal and external factors influence the outcome of a campaign. If successful in obtaining the goal, there will be more work to do following the celebration. The new policy should be continuously reviewed and enhanced, as legislation can be overturned or watered down by other policies, making it much more difficult to enact changes in the future.

If the policy was not adopted, the group should reassemble to go through the original plan and determine areas for improvement. There are always lessons to be learned (e.g., which legislators are adamantly opposed to the issue, better ways to run meetings and communicate with members, which strategies were most effective and least effective). It is important to build on the positives of the campaign, especially if the group was able to mobilize community members around the issue, and provide them with strategies for implementing legislation. This analysis can provide insight on how to tackle the issue from a better angle.

CONCLUSION

The key premise of this chapter is citizenry involvement. Without it, citizens are mere observers of a "democratic" society. Legislators want, and need to know how their constituents feel about legislative issues in order to be true representatives of the people. Involvement in the legislative process for each group is unique, depending on its membership, goals and objectives, and the political atmosphere of the era. The principles presented in this chapter will hopefully be seen as helpful suggestions to be tested in each community. There are thousands of issues that need legislative attention, and not every one of them can be addressed. Advocacy groups, facilitated by a knowledgeable health educator, must carefully choose which legislative issues are deemed most worthy by the community, and which are most likely to be impacted by legislative advocacy efforts.

References

1.   Michigan Department of Public Health. (1994). *Preparing your policy campaigns*. Lansing, MI: Author.

2.   The Marin Institute for Prevention of Alcohol and Other Drug Problems. (1994). *Advocating for policy change*. San Rafael, CA: Author.

3.   *Webster's Ninth New Collegiate Dictionary*. (1989). Springfield, MA: Merriam-Webster.

4.   Michigan State Legislative Council (1995). *A citizen's guide to state government*. Lansing, MI: Allied Printing.

5.   Americans for Nonsmokers' Rights. (1994). *Tips for testifying*. Berkeley, CA: Author.

6.   Americans for Nonsmokers' Rights. (1994). *Meeting with elected officials*. Berkeley, CA: Author.

7.   ASSIST. (1993). *ASSIST training materials, volume VI: Media advocacy: A strategic tool for change*.

Chapter 10

MEDIA AND ADVOCACY TOOLS

Mary T. Gustas, Ed. Spec.
Lisa E. J. Clark, B.S.

Authors' Comments: *Knowing how to effectively work with the media is not something that happens overnight, but rather evolves over time with practice. The experiences we have gained through working with the media has provided us with opportunities to develop and streamline techniques and style. By understanding how the media works, we have been able to work more cooperatively with media contacts. It is our wish that this chapter provides the reader with insight and an understanding of the intricacies associated with the media. We hope that the information presented in this chapter will positively impact the reader's ability to successfully work with the media.*

Even though our agency is small (three full-time employees), we develop and fax at least four public service announcements and one news release per month to over 175 West Michigan area radio and television stations, newspapers, magazines, and community newsletters. In addition, we receive numerous requests for interviews pertaining to many safety-related issues. With the experiences we have gained through the years, we can honestly say that the media truly can "make or break" an organization.

INTRODUCTION

The three chapters that precede this one deal with issues associated with marketing, media advocacy, and legislative processes. Each chapter highlighted approaches and steps associated with effectively implementing marketing or advocacy campaigns. Many of the media methods and tools used in these approaches are the same. Therefore, the purpose of this chapter is to provide technical skills for the application of tools that are commonly used in marketing and advocacy strategies. In particular, this chapter focuses on how to develop and use public service announcements, news releases, action alerts, fact sheets, interviewing skills, and press kits.

This chapter also focuses on tips and techniques for effectively working with the press and media. Not only is it important to understand how to develop materials, it is imperative to know how to effectively promote these to the press and media.

PUBLIC SERVICE ANNOUNCEMENTS

Public service announcements (PSAs) are short informational announcements typically used by charity, nonprofit, and community organizations. They are designed to be used on the radio or television to educate the public, promote programs or services, and provide resources for behavior or community change. Being one of the most commonly used means of conveying messages to the public, almost all agencies have, at one time or another, developed and used PSAs in their programming efforts. Because most PSAs are relatively easy to produce and use, it has become a standard means for agencies to communicate messages to the public.

There are basically two types of PSAs—those aired on radio and those that appear on television. Of the two, radio announcements are usually much easier to develop, cost less, and have a greater likelihood of being aired. A radio PSA consists of a message, which is less than 60 seconds in length, typed on a double-spaced, 8.5 x 11-inch sheet of paper (see Figures 10-1 and 10-2 for sample PSAs). Included in the PSA are the following:

- *Source.* Who is sending the announcement? Both the individual and the organization should be identified. The name of the organization, city, state, and zip code should be located at the top of the first page.

- *Contact person.* Who is the contact person? This person may be different than the source. Included should be the individual's name, title, and phone number. An e-mail address and fax number may also be useful.

- *Release date and time.* When does this information need to be announced? Is there a particular date when it should be used? For example, a PSA about Labor Day travel should be broadcast at the start of the weekend through the day following Labor Day. A time range should be included if the PSA is designed to be aired at a specific time of day. For instance, some PSAs may be more appropriate if aired during the late-afternoon when adolescents are out of school or workers are commuting home.

Television PSAs are either components of broader state and national campaigns, or developed locally by the agency. Obviously, the PSA that has already been developed is much easier and less costly to use than one that needs to be created from scratch. Usually, these PSAs can be tailored to include a message at the end identifying local contacts and action. In contrast, the advantage to developing a PSA is the personalization of the issue to specific community needs, populations, and problems.

Figure 10-1. Sample Public Service Announcement

Public Service Announcements for the Month of February

FROM: Jack Jones, Community Educator
       Alcohol Awareness Associates
       1323 Turn Lane
       Grand Rapids, MI 49503
       (616) 949-5344

RELEASE DATE: February 18, 1998

TIME: 45 seconds

21 to 34-Year Old Drinking and Driving is on the Rise

RECENTLY RELEASED STATISTICS FROM THE NATIONAL HIGHWAY TRAFFIC SAFETY ADMINISTRATION CONFIRMED DEVASTATING NEWS FROM 1995. FOR THE FIRST TIME LAST YEAR, DRUNK DRIVING STATISTICS ACTUALLY ROSE. DEATHS AND INJURIES HAVE BEEN STEADILY DECLINING FOR THE LAST DECADE . . . UNTIL NOW.

THE DATA DEMONSTRATE THAT DRINKING AND DRIVING AMONG YOUNG ADULTS CONTINUES TO BE A MAJOR PROBLEM. INDIVIDUALS BETWEEN THE AGES 21 TO 34 YEARS ARE RESPONSIBLE FOR MORE ALCOHOL-RELATED FATAL CRASHES THAN ANY OTHER AGE GROUP. THIRTY-FIVE PERCENT OF FATAL COLLISIONS AMONG THIS GROUP ARE ALCOHOL-RELATED. OCCASIONAL IMPAIRED DRIVING IS NOT ACCEPTABLE. RESPONSIBLE DRIVING SHOULD BE A CONSISTENT BEHAVIOR.

- ALWAYS BE RESPONSIBLE WHEN CONSUMING ALCOHOL.
- ANY AMOUNT OF ALCOHOL IN YOUR SYSTEM MAY BE IMPAIRING.
- ALWAYS USE DESIGNATED DRIVERS IF YOU ARE DRINKING.
- A PERSON WHO PREVENTS OTHERS FROM DRINKING AND DRIVING SHOULD BE COMMENDED.

-END-

Some PSAs are designed to invoke an emotional response in the listener or viewer. In these situations, material to be included must elicit the desired response. In comparison, other PSAs may be more cognitively focused, informing listeners of dates and times of events, which would be less dependent on emotional response.

Broadcast stations are interested in airing PSAs for a number of reasons. First, the Federal Communications Commission (FCC) considers a station's public service when deciding whether to review its license. Stations that have provided an adequate amount of free air time, in the interest of the public, have a greater likelihood of license renewal.

Second, most local stations are interested in airing information about events and issues that directly impact the local community. Many of their listeners reside within their community and have a desired interest in activities and issues that directly impact them. For instance, many community members rely heavily on radio and television to inform them of free cholesterol screening, health fairs, and the like. As stations compete for listeners, they have an expressed interest in airing PSAs that are both appealing and informative to their listeners or viewers. PSAs reduce the need for stations to seek out and keep track of community event dates.

Lastly, some stations are interested in PSAs because they usually focus on messages that promote positive health and discourage negative actions. As a major means of communicating information, television and radio stations have an unspoken responsibility to the public for providing avenues that will improve the well-being of society.

Time is a precious commodity in broadcasting. Because time is revenue, every second is tracked. Typically, time blocks are available in 10, 15,

Figure 10-2. Sample Public Service Announcement

FROM: Jean Richards, Community Educator
　　　　　Community Safety Partners
　　　　　1224 Jefferson
　　　　　Kalamazoo, MI 49001
　　　　　(616) 555-3000

RELEASE DATE: December 1, 1998

TIME: 30 seconds

Zip-Zero-Zilch

JUST ONE DRINK BEFORE DRIVING CAN GET YOU BUSTED. YOUNG ADULTS MAY THINK THEY KNOW EVERYTHING ABOUT DRINKING AND DRIVING, BUT DO THEY KNOW THE "ZIP-ZERO-ZILCH" LAW? THIS LAW STATES THAT IF YOU'RE STOPPED, YOU'LL BE TESTED FOR ALCOHOL LEVELS. IF YOU REFUSE THE TEST, YOUR LICENSE IS CUT UP ON THE SPOT AND GONE FOR SIX MONTHS. IF THE TEST SHOWS YOU'VE BEEN DRINKING EVEN ONE BEER, YOU'LL LOSE YOUR LICENSE FOR 30 TO 90 DAYS AND PAY UP TO $250 IN FINES.

IN MICHIGAN, THE ONLY WAY YOU CAN DRIVE SAFELY IS IF YOU HAVE HAD "ZIP-ZERO-ZILCH" TO DRINK.

THIS MESSAGE IS BROUGHT TO YOU BY COMMUNITY SAFETY PARTNERS.

-END-

20, 30, 45, and 60-second lengths. The longer 60-second spots are typically reserved for well-known agencies, such as the American Red Cross or United Way. Most PSAs, however, span a 30-second or less time block.

Prior to writing the PSA, all information pertaining to the topic should be gathered and organized in a fashion to which it is easy to refer. Because the PSA is rather short in length, material to be included will have to be carefully selected. The PSA needs to be written in a concise manner. This may be difficult at first because this is a skill that is not often used in an academic setting. Having colleagues and members of the target audience proofread the PSA will improve the quality of the piece. Reading the copy aloud while timing it will assist in determining the length. When doing so, however, it is important to read at the same pace at which the PSA will appear on the radio or television. Timing does not have to be exact, however, as the station staff will trim the copy to fit their time. Usually, the station will call if they need further information.

The PSA should be sent or faxed, along with a cover letter explaining the importance of the announcement, to targeted stations. Because stations receive volumes of PSA requests, they should be submitted early so that air time can be scheduled. It is recommended that submissions occur at least six weeks prior to the announcement date.

Some organizations have access to technological resources that can produce video and audio PSAs. These should also be held to a 30-second spot. If they are received from a national resource, it is usually possible to request that they be customized to identify the local contact. This should be addressed in the cover letter accompanying the material. If there are only a few stations that will be receiving the material, it would be advantageous to call and inform them of the material being sent.

NEWS RELEASES

Conventional news, or press, releases provide information about an organization and its activities. They are designed to be used by radio, television, newspapers, or regional/local magazines. For example, an organization could use this technique to announce new board or staff members or a special activity. This tool is often used by an organization to gain community recognition for their organization, activities, or members (see Figures 10-3 and 10-4 for sample news releases).

The news release is a one or two page double spaced typed document (8.5 x 11-inch). In addition to the source, contact person and release date and time, the release needs to include the following:

- *Headline.* The headline provides the overall concept of the information and should be typed in capital letters. Headlines can be up to three lines long, but keeping them to one or two lines is more effective. Without the headline, the media will take it upon themselves to decide what it should be labeled. Allowing this to happen may be detrimental, especially if they make a mistake and misinterpret the content.

- *Story.* The story is the content of the news release and can be one of two types—a news story or a feature. A news story provides information about an announcement or is an account of an activity that readers may find of interest. Figures 10-3 and 10-4 represent sample news stories. In contrast, a feature is a story that is a main attraction or head liner. For instance, a news release pertaining to a breakthrough in Cancer research from the National Institutes of Health or a disease epidemic from the Centers for Disease Control and Prevention are front page news (see Figure 10-5 for sample feature story news release).

  In a news story, the first paragraph is the most important. It must contain the basics of journalism: Who, what, where, and when. Be prepared to have the rest of the story cut by an editor. Because newsprint and air time is limited, it is best to follow an inverted triangle in writing the news story. With an inverted tri-

Figure 10-3. Sample News Release

FROM: American First Aid
        123 Eagle Drive
        Northport, MI 49670

CONTACT: Bill Waiter

PHONE: (312) 456-2367

FAX: (312) 763-2654

DATE: February 10, 1998

                                        FOR IMMEDIATE RELEASE

               FREE FIRST AID/CPR TRAINING AVAILABLE

The American First Aid Institute announced today a promotional "buy one get one free" First Aid/CPR training, as part of their grand opening. A total of 10 training programs, each limited to 12 individuals, will be available. Each training will be conducted over an 8-hour day, beginning on Saturday, August 30.
    Enrollment is on a first-come basis. For more information or to register for the class, call (312) 456-2367 or stop by American First Aid at 123 Eagle Drive.

                                XXX

Figure 10-4. Sample News Release

FROM: Bobbin Funeral Home
        51 Michigan Avenue
        Milwaukee, WI

CONTACT: Bill Hobbit, Jr.

PHONE: (612) 767-4763

FAX: (612) 767-4764

FOR IMMEDIATE RELEASE

FREE SEMINAR: GRIEF MANAGEMENT

Milwaukee, WI - Bobbin Funeral Home is sponsoring a free seminar on "Grief Management." Speaking will be the internationally recognized author on separation and loss, Gaylord Kane. The primary audience for this session, which will be held on Friday, November 18 at noon, includes care givers in health and human services professions. This program will be held at Discovery Theatre, 200 Michigan Ave. Call (612) 767-4763 to reserve a seat.

END

---

angle, the most important sentence is listed first followed by the next most important and so on. If the story is to be cut, chances are that the editor will cut the bottom portion, where the least important information is contained.

If the story is a feature, it will need to contain more information within the body. Features are also edited, but are written more to gain the attention of the editor and draw them into the entire text. The objective of the feature is to get the entire story printed. Unfortunately, this is not always the case.

Triple spacing should be used between the headline and the first paragraph of the story. Paragraphs should not be split between pages. If there is a chance a paragraph may continue on to the subsequent page, the entire paragraph should be moved to the next page. Consider if each paragraph can stand alone with or without the previous or following paragraph. If the release is designed to solicit a response, contact information needs to be in the last paragraph (e.g., "For more information, please contact Greg Shelley at (800) 212-4620").

- *Closing.* Typing "END," "###," or "XXX" at the end of the story text identifies the end of the release to the editor.

Figure 10-5. Sample Feature Story Press Release

FROM: Center for Disease Control
        Atlanta, GA

CONTACT: Michael Haines, M.D., Ph.D.

PHONE: (412) 232-3432

FAX: (412) 232-2654

DATE: February 10, 1998

FOR IMMEDIATE RELEASE

EBOLA VIRUS THREATENS LIVES IN ZIMBABWE

Atlanta, GA - The Centers for Disease Control and Prevention announced today that the threat of the ebola virus in Zimbabwe has reached epidemic proportions. To date, over 325,000 people have contracted the disease. Death usually results within 48 hours of infection. Immunologists are working around the clock to find a vaccine. With infections continuing at the current rate, the expected death toll may reach over one million. All travel to Zimbabwe should be avoided, if possible. Any shipments that have been received over the past 20 days must be maintained in quarantine until further notice.

    If anyone is aware of individuals or packages that have recently arrived from Zimbabwe, contact the Centers for Disease Control and Prevention immediately at (800) 363-7462. Calls will be answered 24 hours a day, seven days a week.

XXX

There are a number of ways to increase the likelihood that the release will be published:

- Keep the press release short. Make each sentence concise and avoid using jargon.

- Provide the media with a detailed fact sheet as a supplement.

- Format facts to stand independently from the release. This will also eliminate "clutter."

- Write the press release so that it does not need a cover letter to explain the contents.

- Allow for wide margins and double spaces. This is called white space. It provides editors with room need for editing.

- Write the news release in a professional manner. This will increase respect from the media.

ACTION ALERTS

Action alerts are designed to motivate a targeted recipient to take action on a specific issue. Agencies, lobbying groups, charities and other organizations use action alerts to notify their affiliates, supporters, state and federal elected officials, or board members.

The action alert is not used for any specific issues or circumstances. Its purpose is to secure an immediate response from a targeted group. The alert may provide information regarding pending legislation, unequal treatment, an upcoming vote, or some other item that requires support or action. Material contained in the alert may be several pages long or just a few paragraphs. It provides the recipient with the explanation of the pending activity and the needed support or participation on their part. Usually included are a response date, phone numbers to call, addresses to write letters, and a time, date and location for a rally or demonstration. The action alert may take the form of a letter, fax, or even a phone call (see Figures 10-6 and 10-7 for sample action alerts).

MEDIA AND LEGISLATIVE FACT SHEETS

Media fact sheets are tools used to secure feature articles in a newspaper or magazine. Members of the media do not always investigate or seek out stories based on their own interests. Most articles are a result of some impetus provided from a reliable source. The fact sheet is sent to the media for encouragement and consideration for further investigation, perhaps to be used in a feature story. It may also be referred to as a background paper (see Figure 10-8 for sample media fact sheet).

The fact sheet is very different from a PSA or news release in that it provides a structured format of information to the editor for assistance in developing a story idea. It does not provide all the details of the story, but rather plants a seed for an idea that can be expanded into a longer, more detailed article. From the information presented in the fact sheet, the editor will determine if a writer should be assigned the topic to develop a follow-up article.

The legislative fact sheet serves a similar purpose but is targeted toward impacting legislation. It is used to educate legislators or citizens about an area of concern or interest and provides background information on items that are, or might be, acted upon by legislators. For instance, an effort could be made to convince legislators that a particular law should not be repealed or should be introduced. This same information may later be used to convince voters to take a similar position (see Figure 10-9 for sample legislative fact sheet). Legislative aides may be assigned to more thoroughly research the topic or issue. In doing so, they perform similar research to that of a reporter in developing a news article. In particular, the aide may conduct interviews and perhaps actually write a position paper or draft legislation for submission by the legislator.

Figure 10-6. Sample Action Alert

ACTION ALERT

TO: Wai Ki Ki Surfers Association

FROM: Aloha, Inc.

RE: HB 2304

DATE: April 23, 1997

Aloha, Inc. urges you to contact (by phone, fax, letter, or e-mail) the following legislators, all of whom serve on the Water Safety Subcommittee, and urge them to vote against HB 2304æa bill that requires surfers to wear protective helmets during all water activity. This bill is currently in committee and expected to be reviewed on May 1, 1997.

Name	Phone	Fax
Rep. John Brown (Chair)	(555) 123-3355	(555) 123-3352
Rep. Martha Smots	(555) 123-4353	(555) 123-4354
Rep. Tim Turton	(555) 123-3272	(555) 123-3273
Rep. Perk Sonnega	(555) 123-5782	(555) 123-5783
Rep. Rodney Prahl	(555) 123-4456	(555) 123-4457

Letters may be sent to:

Honorable _____
House of Representatives
4040 Skylark
Honolulu, HI 91432

It is just a matter of time until all water activities are curtailed by legislation such as this. We believe it would be foolish to enact such legislation for the following reasons:

- Water helmets have been proven to increase serious injuries to the wearer, particularly in high wake situations.

- Water helmets currently have no regulations regarding safety specifications.

- The use of water helmets will greatly reduce the tourism to the Hawaiian Islands.

- Mandatory use of water helmets is an infringement of personal choice.

Thank you for your support in this important issue.

###

Most of the time, a cover letter should accompany the media or legislative fact sheet. The letter should not be wordy or reflect a desperate plea for consideration, but rather a brief summary of the basic concept, description of the problem, and possible solutions. Additional information can include the name of a key contact person who is available for an interview and an explanation of the importance the issue has to a broader audience.

Fact sheets should include:

- *Source.* Who is the legislative or media fact sheet from? Both the individual and the organization need to be identified. Name and address should be located at the top left hand corner of the page.

- *Contact person.* Who is the contact person responsible for answering questions related to the fact sheet?

Figure 10-7. Sample Action Alert

ACTION ALERT

TO: All Members of the Christian Action Force

FROM: Rev. Jackson Holliday
    My Home Church
    1356 Beech

RE: Neighborhood Children's Watch

DATE: August 20, 1997

On Sunday, August 28, 1997, My Home Church will be sponsoring a speak-out against Children's Violence. The program will be held in the church parking lot, located at 1436 Washington, Chicago, IL.

Your presence is requested to show support for this very important issue. Over the past 16 months in Chicago, there have been numerous acts of violence targeted toward children under the age of 14.

The following individuals will be present to speak in support of this issue:

    3:45 PM Rev. Jackson Holliday - Opening remarks
    4:00 PM Oprah Winfrey
    4:45 PM Mayor Dailey
    5:00 PM Michael Jordan
    5:30 PM Police Chief Jackson
    6:00 PM Rev. Jackson Holliday - Closing comments

It is important that we show how much we care about the children of this city. Thank you for caring enough to be there for them.

###

Figure 10-8. Sample Media Fact Sheet

FROM: Baby Safety Center
        2020 Congress (202) 625-BABY
        Washington, DC 20000

CONTACT: Nancy Newsworthy

FACT SHEET: Air Bags And Safety Belts

The Purpose of Air Bags:
- Air bags are designed to decrease head and chest injuries in frontal impact crashes. They are not designed to replace safety belts but to provide additional protection to the occupants of motor vehicles.

Benefits of Air Bags:
- Air bags have saved over 2,000 lives since being required in passenger vehicles.
- Air bags have reduces fatalities in 30% of head-on crashes.
- Automobile injuries have dropped 24% since air bags have been introduced.

Risks of Air Bags:
- Air bags inflate at an estimated rate of 200 m.p.h..
- Thirty-two deaths, primarily involving children, have been related to air bag deployment on the passenger side.

Solutions:
- Infants should never ride on the passenger side of a vehicle with a passenger air bag system.
- Children under 12 should always ride in the back seat with proper safety belt restraints.
- Drivers should always obey speed limits.

Included should be the person's name, title, phone number and extension. This information is also located at the top left hand corner of the page.

- *Title.* Following a triple space appears the capitalized title "FACT SHEET." A subtitle can be listed after the fact sheet heading.

- *Body.* This section consists of the specific information that is related to the topic.

INTERVIEWS

The media may be interested in obtaining further information via a telephone, radio, or television interview, especially if a relationship between the agency and the media already exists. Periodically, the news releases,

Figure 10-9. Sample Legislative Fact Sheet

FROM: Community Safety Partners
        555 Lane Blvd.
        Kalamazoo, MI 49000
        (616) 555-3000

CONTACT: Suzie Kurn

LEGISLATIVE FACT SHEET: Administrative License Revocation

- Administrative License Revocation (ALR) allows any arresting officer to confiscate the driving license of an individual who is legally intoxicated or refuses to take a blood-alcohol concentration test.

- The officer will usually issue a temporary driving permit that is valid for a limited time. The offender may appeal the revocation through an administrative hearing.

- If the driver does not appeal or if the revocation is upheld, the offender loses driving privileges for a set period.

- Impaired drivers may lose their license in states with no ALR laws, but only after a criminal court conviction. Often due to considerable "red tape," an offender's license may never be revoked.

ALR works because drivers who are arrested and have their licenses revoked under ALR are less likely to drink and drive again. ALR has proven to be preventative in discouraging people from driving while impaired because it causes them to worry about losing their licenses if they do drink and drive.

---

action alerts, PSAs, or media fact sheets that are disseminated result in a request for an interview. The interview can be either formal or more relaxed. It may be conducted over the phone, on-site at the radio or television station, at the interviewee's agency, or at some other off-site location. Regardless of the location or medium, it is best to always be prepared for an interview. Because of their widespread ability to reach masses, media calls should always take top priority.

In general, reporters can be very demanding. When they call, their deadline for material is usually extremely tight. Maintaining a good relationship with the media requires being flexible and accommodating to their schedule. Cooperating with their demands may result in additional interviews in the future.

Telephone Interview

A telephone interview is initiated with a call requesting an interview or statement related to a particular news item. Prior to engaging in the interview, a number of points must be considered:

- Make sure that the agency does not have a policy on public relations that states only certain individuals can talk to the press.

- Determine who is calling and the topic of inquiry.

- Do not hesitate to take a moment to gather background information or offer to call back when the information has been obtained. This allows an opportunity to review the material prior to responding to the interviewer's questions. If the interview is a result of a PSA, news release, fact sheet or action alert, most questions will either reiterate what has already been written, or will clarify an item within the material.

- Remain calm and professional. Nervous reactions are likely to be recognized over the phone and on the radio.

Telephone interviewers usually have prepared questions and are ready to guide individuals through the process. Some telephone interviews will come from radio stations that want another voice to be heard on the air. These interviews may be taped. If so, mistakes can be made as they will be edited later. Other times the interview will be a live broadcast. Regardless, the organization needs to be recognized and a phone number provided for additional information.

Radio Interviews

Some radio stations have talk shows or community information sessions. If called to participate in a radio interview, the following should be considered:

- Know who will be conducting the interview. If not familiar with the person, listen to the show prior to the interview. Become familiar with and understand the format and interview style.

- Who listens to the show? Is the audience primarily (e.g.) teens, elderly, high income, or highly educated? Audience information may be available from the marketing department of the radio station or from discussions with people who are familiar with the program.

- Prepare to answer as many questions as possible. Some stations will provide a sample of questions that will be asked. Other questions, however, may come up in the conversation or from callers.

- Make a list of the major points you want to relay. If the host does not ask for the information, try to add it into the conversation.

- State the organization's address or phone number as often as possible.

- Do not be afraid to take organized reference material with you. The key term is organize—shuffling through papers is not a positive image. As it is hard to remember everything, being able to locate information quickly is a benefit. These materials are particularly important if the show allows for call-in questions.

- Do not be afraid to say "That is a good question. I do not know the answer off the top of my head. I will have to do some additional research and get back to you." Admitting lack of knowledge is much better than providing inaccurate or incorrect information.

- Have a final statement prepared. Typically, the host will ask if there is anything else to add. Take advantage of the opportunity to advertise the agency or make a significant statement about the topic.

- Do not be late. Remember time is a precious commodity for both radio and television.

Television Interviews

Television interviews are slightly different than telephone or radio interviews. In some situations, interview requests are made in advance. Other times the interview may need to be conducted within the hour in response to a news item that just come over the wire. In both of these situations, prepared information may not be readily available. Having an organized filing system allows quick access to background information. It may be necessary to become an expert on an area fairly quickly. If, for some reason, it is not possible to be interviewed, the station needs to be informed and provided with other possible resources.

Suggestions for enhancing the interview include the following:

- Look your best. Clean shirt, tie, polished shoes, nice dress, and groomed. Imagine the President of the United States is in the audience.

- Take time to prepare for questions.

- Selected apparel should be conservative and medium gray, browns, khaki, or blue. Avoid wild patterns or stripes. The clothing selection is important for at least two reasons: (1) A professional representation is important, and (2) clashing with the television set is not helpful in relaying a message.

- Accessories should be limited to a watch and ring. Do not over-use accessories that may glare or reflect in the lights. In addition, do not use accessories that make noise (e.g., some jewelry). Wear glasses if they are usually worn.

- Maintain good posture. Sit comfortably in the chair but do not slouch. Keep legs crossed or feet flat on the floor and lean slightly forward toward the interviewer. Do not gesture with hand movements. Make sure hands remain above the waist.

Interviews are also requested at the spur of the moment. If the media requests an immediate interview, there is little time to enhance professional appearance. If usually dressed casually, it is a good idea to have accessories that can provide a professional touch. For example, men can keep a pressed shirt and tie on-site. Women could keep a blazer and nice blouse hanging in the corner.

Last minute interview requests require an expert to respond. When contacted by the media, the topic of the interview and how long the interview will last needs to be determined. If unfamiliar with the subject, it is acceptable to decline the interview as long as the interview is not related to an agency position or other relevant issue. Never leave the press in a position to make assumptions about sensitive or relevant issues such as clarifying an agency's position. There is a reason for wanting to conduct the interviews in the first place. They want to report factual information, not assumptions.

A business card that identifies the organization, phone number, contact name, and title should be brought to the interview. If additional background information is available on the interview topic, copies can be provided to the reporter. Good interview can be shaped by providing additional background information to reporters as they may only have a small amount of information that appeared on a fact sheet from the wire service. Most reporters are very thankful for the information because it saves research time.

The interview may take an hour or more and result in only 15 seconds on the air. Even so, 15 seconds on the 6:00 or 11:00 o'clock news may result in many phone calls. If an interviewer does call, be prepared to answer phone questions and send appropriate materials if requested by a listener.

PRESS KITS

The press kit is a packet of prepared information about a particular topic, story, or event, that is provided to the media and other interested agencies.

Press kits are typically prepared when a press conference is scheduled or special event planned such as a political rally or other public news session. For instance, a press kit could be developed for the opening of a new museum or library, or in conjunction with the release of the latest local statistics on AIDS and Hepatitis by the local community health department. Ensuring the same information is disseminated to all interested parties eliminates the need for individual interviews or extra copying of materials. In addition, by providing the material to the press and media, better control maintained over the information released.

The material found in the press kit is pre-written and can include public relations material used for other events. Press kits provide the media and other interested parties with answers to questions that arise related to the organization or the topic. Not having a press kit available for a special event or press conference may result in extra work in preparing responses and fulfilling requests for information.

Press kits are usually presented in pocket folders and prepared in a visually appealing manner. Having an impressive folder portrays a positive image of the organization. Some organizations, though, present the material in an expensive glossy package in an attempt to impress the media. This is wasteful as reporters determine the value of information on content, not presentation. This is not to say that low quality is desired. The folder should be impressive but still cost effective.

Contents of a Press Kit

Technically, almost anything can be included in a press kit. There are no specific rules or regulations the media requires or has designated as most appropriate. Some items that are beneficial include the following:

- *Kit cover.* This is the actual folder in which the material is presented. An imprint or label with the organization's logo is a must. Adding a headline about the contents may also be beneficial.

- *Organization information sheet.* This provides background on the organization that is holding the press conference or special event. It is particularly helpful if the organization is not well known or fairly new. Information sheets may be presented in a booklet format. The information on these sheets includes agency services, locations, financial information, key achievements, research activities, community activities, awards, mission statements, and goals and objectives.

- *Biographical statements.* The press should be provided with information on the qualifications of those speaking at the event. This information lends credibility to the presenter. Included should be the presenter's full name, job title, responsibilities, degrees, publications, accomplishments, and memberships. Length should be no more than a half to a full page.

- *Fact sheet.* The fact sheet consists of background information on the topic being presented. It should not be detailed but written so that it highlights important facts related to the issue. The purpose is to give a quick overview of the subject. The use of bullets, tables, graphs or numbers is completely acceptable. The fact sheet should be between one to three pages (see Figures 10-8 and 10-9 for sample fact sheets).

- *Photographs.* Photos may be of the speaker(s), products, or featured event. Photographs should be black and white and at least 5 x 7-inches in size. A label written with a fine-point felt marker can be posted on the back of the picture.

- *Article reprints.* If the topic has received previous press coverage, it is beneficial to provide copies of the articles in the press kit. This provides additional credibility to the topic for its newsworthiness.

- *Catalogs and brochures.* The agency may have other products or services that it would like to present. The press kit serves as an avenue to advertise these items. Discretion needs to be used to avoid overloading the press kit with materials that have little to do with the press conference or event.

- *Public announcement.* If a speech is associated with the presentation of the press kit, a copy of the prepared announcement should be included. This assists media representatives in obtaining accurate quotes, spelling of names, and references.

CONCLUSION

Each of the tools presented in this chapter may be used in any community health education agency with some more applicable than others. The tools assist in bringing an awareness of inappropriate social behavior that should be changed in order to ensure a safer and healthier life. Typically, attitudes are not changed as a result of media tools, because most attitudes are deeply rooted within the social culture. An effective PSA or news release, however, may increase awareness and initiate a questioning process in individuals. Both legislators and the public can be influenced through the use of appropriate media tools. In general, to significantly impact a legislative change, lobbying and door-to-door canvassing must accompany the prepared materials. None of the activities presented in this and other chapters will succeed in changing behaviors on their own. Consistent use and development of positive working relations with the press and media increases the likelihood of impacting change.

Chapter 11

PRINTED EDUCATIONAL MATERIALS

Stephanie Sikora, B.S., C.H.E.S.

Author's Comments: *Being creative is probably the biggest asset needed for developing printed health education materials. The development of printed materials, however, is no longer just for graphic designers. For instance, I never used to consider myself to be an exceptionally creative person, but with practice, I have found that creativity can be developed with patience and experimentation. The key thing to remember is it takes time to learn what does and does not work. I have learned a great deal by watching other people, and reviewing pamphlets and materials that have already been developed. Of course, much of what I am attracted to is driven by my own personal taste. Most readers, however, are attracted to similar things, like simplicity, relevance, and attractiveness.*

The ideas presented in this chapter are guidelines. There are no rules when developing printed educational materials. What works well for one piece may not work for another. Professional preparation programs do not necessarily prepare individuals to develop effective printed educational materials. Throughout college, I strove to develop my writing skills to a high reading level. Upon entering the health education field, I really was not prepared to write at a sixth grade reading level again. It takes hard work and patience to write for a variety of audiences, but I have found that developing printed educational materials is one of my favorite things to do.

INTRODUCTION

People require different modes of "input" in order to retain and learn new information. Presenting materials visually is one such method. As a health educator, it is often necessary to develop printed materials to enhance or supplement other educational strategies. Often, people are intimidated by asking questions. Printed materials can provide information they need, but are too afraid to ask. In addition, printed educational materials reinforce messages from other sources and provide an excellent means for disseminating information about resources that are available on health related topics.

The development of printed educational materials is a time-consuming and arduous process that should not be taken lightly. It may seem like a simple task to develop a printed piece such as a newsletter, pamphlet, or flyer. However, if information is to be understood, retained, and utilized for behavior change, it must be appropriate, interesting, simple, and necessary. The difficult task is making all elements of the piece fall within these guides. For example, if the cover or heading does not grab the reader's attention immediately, the individual may choose not to read any further. As with any health education program development, a health education programming model can be applied to the development of printed educational materials.

10-STEP PLANNING MODEL

Health educators are accustomed to following a series of steps to ensure successful programming. The same steps can be applied to the development of printed educational materials. Planning, implementation, and evaluation have been recognized as critical components of the health education process. By following the same steps for material development, health educators will write and produce the best piece possible. The following 10 steps for program planning can be applied to the development of printed education materials.[1]

1. Define the General Idea or Main Purpose

Prior to beginning the development of any printed educational piece, there must be a predefined purpose for doing so. The need for developing the product may be due to (1) requests for unavailable materials, (2) the results of a needs assessment, (3) available materials are out-of-date or inappropriate for a particular audience, (4) available materials are too expensive to purchase, or (5) the emergence of a new public health issue.

For example, prior to 1981, AIDS was not a public health issue in the U.S. In fact, the term AIDS was unknown to most physicians, let alone the general public. Today, HIV and AIDS are acronyms familiar to nearly every household. The widespread distribution of printed educational materials, in addition to other educational strategies, is directly responsible for the rapid increase in HIV / AIDS awareness.

2. Complete an Assessment and Evaluation of the Organization, Resources, Regulations, and Policies

Once an idea has been recognized, an internal assessment of resources should occur. During this process, the following questions need to be considered:

- Will administration allow the project to be done?

- Will the community accept and support the project?

- Are there any legal issues to be addressed?

- Are the necessary resources (e.g., computers, copiers, finances, paper, printers, staff, and expertise) available to proceed?

- Are there any regulations or policies that need to be taken into consideration?

Regulations and policies may affect information that is included within a printed piece. For instance, in some school districts the word "condom" cannot be mentioned. This has a major impact on what HIV/AIDS and pregnancy prevention materials can be distributed to youth.

3. Develop Goals and Objectives for the Needs Assessment

Prior to implementing a needs assessment, it is important to identify what is to be accomplished. Setting goals and objectives for a needs assessment will aid in the development of an effective assessment tool. The following questions should be addressed by these goals and objectives:

- What is the purpose of the needs assessment?

- Who will conduct the needs assessment?

- What is the time line for completion of the needs assessment?

- Who will evaluate the results of the needs assessment?

- What format will be used for the assessment? A survey? Focus groups?

4. Conduct a Needs Assessment

In order to develop materials that are appropriate for a target audience, the author must conduct extensive research pertinent to that group. Assumptions should never be made. For example, in an HIV/AIDS pamphlet, the term "partner" may be more appropriate than "husband" or "boyfriend." The more closely the audience can be defined, the more successful the pamphlet will be at increasing awareness and impacting behavior change. A needs assessment will also assist the health educator in determining which audience to target. The following questions are pertinent to a needs assessment:

- Are existing materials already available?

- What are the inadequacies and strengths of existing materials?

- What cultural issues need to be addressed?

- What gaps are there in current knowledge?

- What is the literacy level of the intended audience?

- What information is appropriate for the group? (e.g., it would not be appropriate to tell a group of second graders about cleaning a needle or syringe to prevent HIV transmission)

- What are the cultural attitudes and beliefs surrounding the topic?

- What barriers exist for the target audience?

Culture plays an especially important role in health beliefs, attitudes, and behaviors. For instance, printed health material that is successful with one population may be perceived by a different population as unattractive, incomprehensible, or contrary to their cultural beliefs.[2] Involving the target audience from the beginning will help ensure their needs are met.

5. Determine and Set Priorities

Results of the needs assessment will aid in prioritizing what should be included in the printed material. People need to know, "what is in it for me?" Information that the audience "needs to know" should be separated from the information that is "nice to know." For example, if a pamphlet were being developed for injection drug users, information about how to clean needles would take priority over information about "safer sex."

6. Develop Goals and Objectives

Once priority areas have been determined, goals and objectives should be aimed at those areas. The development of goals and objectives is often overlooked, but is crucial for the successful development of printed health education materials. Without clearly defined goals and objectives, the developer is without direction. Goals and objectives should be developed around the main idea or general purpose of the material. In addition, it is important that the goals and objectives be reasonable, attainable, and measurable. For health education materials, they should revolve around the behavior change of the reader (see Table 11-1).

Table 11-1. Sample Goal and Objectives for an HIV / AIDS Pamphlet

---

Goal: The reader will know what to do in order to receive an HIV-antibody test.

Knowledge Objective: At least 80% of readers will be able to state two local HIV-antibody testing sites after reading the pamphlet.

Behavior Objective: At least 25% of readers will get an HIV-antibody test within one year of reading the pamphlet.

Goals and objectives should target information that is "need to know," from that which is "nice to know." Most educational materials are limited in space, and goals and objectives will help the author in making the best use of that space.

7. Step-by-Step Activities and Strategies

After content planning is complete, the development process and layout needs to be considered. The following questions can guide this phase:

- How should the material be presented? (e.g., pamphlet, flyer, monthly newsletter)
- How should the material be laid out?
- Who will be responsible for the computer layout?
- Which computer program will work best for *this* material?
- What graphics should be used?
- How many copies will be printed, by whom, and how much will they cost?
- On what size paper will the material be printed?
- Will the printing be done in black-and-white or color?
- Will people need to be recruited for focus groups or to review the material?

It is helpful to draw a prototype on paper before beginning layout on a computer. For instance, in developing a pamphlet, an 8.5 x 11-inch piece of paper can be folded into thirds and planned for spacing, layout, and organization.

8. Develop a Time Line

The development of educational materials is time consuming. This is especially true when the final product needs to be reviewed and approved by administration or outside parties. A time line should be developed that reflects printing, evaluation, and revisions phases. Additional time needs to be planned for if materials must undergo translation or professional proofing.

9. Develop a "Final Draft" of the Printed Material

Essentially, this step focuses on the development of the final product before evaluation. The development of the final draft involves combining text with graphics using a computer program. Before the piece is evaluated by the target audience, there may be some internal evaluation requirements to consider. The piece may require supervisory or administrative approval. It is important to follow any internal protocols prior to taking the material outside the agency for evaluation.

10. Evaluate Printed Materials

As with any health education program, evaluation is an essential component in the development of effective printed materials. It is especially important when materials are being developed for specific target audiences. If materials are not evaluated and reviewed, it is possible that information will not be retained, understood, or acted upon. Although it may seem unnecessary, an evaluation should always be conducted prior to large-scale printing and distribution. It can prevent the loss of time, money, and valuable resources. The following questions are appropriate for this phase:

- Is the goal being met?
- Are the objectives being met?
- Is the information appropriate for the intended audience?
- Is the reading level appropriate?
- Is the information needed or wanted?

It is possible that some individuals may be offended by the graphics or information contained within a printed piece. For instance, many people are taught to lose weight in order to control their diabetes. Some ethnic groups, however, do not value being slim or small-framed. This is true with some Native-Americans. It would be important to know this when planning what and how information should be included in a brochure targeting Native-Americans. It would be ineffective, and possibly offensive, to design a whole pamphlet around weight loss for Native-Americans. A more effective approach would be to explain in greater detail other prevention strategies than weight loss.

A variety of methods exist for determining whether or not information is appropriate and accurate for a specific audience. Common techniques include (1) proof reading, (2) peer review, (3) field testing, (4) content review, (5) pretest/post-test, and (6) readability index.

Proof Reading

Many strategies exist for proofing text. For instance, reading lines backwards helps identify spelling and punctuation errors that may otherwise be missed. Reading pages in random order also helps point out errors. If time is available, the piece should be read several days after the final draft has been completed. This break will give the writer or proofer enough time to approach the material with a fresh eye. Having others proof the material is always a good way to catch errors.

Peer Review

Printed materials should be reviewed by a group of peers for accuracy, spelling, grammar, and design. Peer review could be conducted by a variety of people such as coworkers, other health educators, and graphic designers. Anyone that has a solid understanding of what makes printed educational materials work would be a good choice. Peer review is an inexpensive and accessible way to evaluate printed materials.

Field Testing

The purpose of field, or pilot testing is to ensure that the target audience is receiving the intended message(s) and retaining the content. Field testing involves administering a short quiz (5-10 questions) to 25 - 50 members of the target audience. Questions should be simple and directly related to the four or five main points pertinent to the material. The quiz is not a test of the reader's intelligence, but rather designed to determine whether or not the typical reader understands the printed material. This method is also referred to as learner verification. Learner verification assures that the reader is learning the information that is intended.

In addition to a content quiz, more general questions should be included. Based on responses, revisions can be made. The following questions are appropriate for a pamphlet:

- What words would you use to describe the pamphlet?

- Do the pictures help you understand the message?

- How could the pamphlet be improved?

- Did the pamphlet provide you with any new information?

- Was there anything that was unclear?

Content Review

Health educators should make every possible effort to verify that the information presented in their printed material is accurate and true. An expert in the content area associated with the printed material should be asked to review the piece for accuracy. For example, it would be appropriate for an oncologist, or representative from the American Cancer Society to review a pamphlet on the topic of skin cancer for accuracy.

Pretest/Post-test

Administering a pretest to members of the target audience, prior to reading the material, measures their current level of knowledge. Results of a post-test can be compared to those of the pretest, indicating increases in knowledge.

Readability

A readability test should be conducted to ensure the material is at an appropriate reading level for the target audience. (A more complete discussion pertaining to readability is presented in the next section of this chapter.)

GUIDELINES FOR DEVELOPING PRINTED MATERIALS

In public health, most printed materials are developed for broad constituencies. Readers come from a variety of cultural and educational backgrounds. Most readers, regardless of their background, can appreciate the ease that good content and design provide. As mentioned earlier, there are no hard and fast rules that apply to writing and producing educational materials. The following guidelines, however, can *aid* in the development of a successful printed piece.

Layout

Layout involves the combination of text and graphics on a page. Readers appreciate a balance between the two. A well-designed layout is done in a way that works for the audience, organizes information, and attracts attention.[3] The following guidelines will aid in the development of an effective layout.

- *Always leave ample white space.* If materials are too crowded, it is difficult for readers to sort through information. It is no wonder then that readers appreciate the use of ample white space (the space on a page not covered with words or graphics). Text should be balanced with graphics, graphical elements (boxes, lines, tables), and white space. White space does not necessarily need to be distributed evenly. In fact, it is sometimes effective to place large blocks of white space together. In other instances, it may be appropriate to use white space more consistently. Do not assume that the entire area *must* be filled (see Figure 11-1).

- *Use bullets and numbering to highlight key points.* Using bulleted or numbered lists makes it easy for readers to identify main ideas without sorting through unnecessary information. Each list should have a simple, instructional heading. Limit lists to five or six items, and if more room is needed, use subheadings. Lists also aid in the presentation of sequential information.

Figure 11-1. Use of White Space

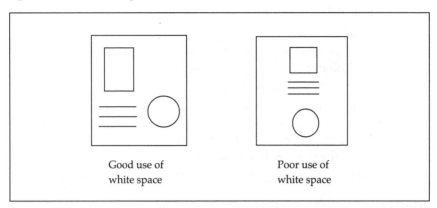

Good use of   Poor use of
white space   white space

- *Set up margins that facilitate easy reading.* Margins should always be equal on the left and right, but not necessarily on top and bottom. Left and right margins should usually be set at .5 or 1 inch. Anything less tends to make the material appear too cluttered and line lengths become too long. Rather than making the top and bottom margins equal, the bottom margin should be the wider of the two to prevent the text from looking top heavy.

- *Use a jagged right edge.* Readers have an easier time reading text with a jagged right edge. Right or full justification makes it difficult for a reader's eyes to follow text down the page. Using right justification against a graphic with a straight left edge, however, provides for a cleaner look.

- *Limit ideas to three or four key points.* During the planning phase, goals and objectives should be prioritized and limited to three or four main points. Trying to fit too much information in any one piece will make it difficult for the reader to retain *any* of the information.

- *Plan materials so that important ideas follow a "Z" pattern.* Most readers are right-eye dominate, meaning they first look at the upper left corner, then move to the upper right, then to the bottom left, and finally to the bottom right of a page. Therefore, the most important idea should be in the upper left and flow to the bottom right corner. Advertisers are very aware of this. For example, the Surgeon General's Warning is required by law to be placed on tobacco billboards and ads. Generally, the warning is placed in the far bottom left corner of the ad, a place where the eye does not normally travel.

- *Use generous spacing.* Single spacing is often difficult to read. As a rule of thumb, multiple-spacing should be used to separate paragraphs.

- *Use horizontal print, rather than vertical.* People are accustomed to reading from left to right across a page. Vertical print can challenge even strong readers.

- *Avoid "orphan" lines.* Orphan lines are those that do not fit on the same page, or in the same column as the rest of the text. The layout should be rearranged so a minimum of two lines are set off by themselves. It is better to move a whole paragraph or section to the next page then to leave a line or two stranded.

Print/Font

Poorly chosen font, style, or size can greatly impair a piece's readability. An abundance of literature is available that describes the intricacies of print and font choices. A few basic guidelines for printed educational materials include the following:

- *Use at least a 12-point type size.* In general, it is best to use either a 12-point or 14-point type size. Larger sizes may be used to highlight main ideas, themes, headings, or titles (see Figure 11-2). Anything smaller is difficult to read. A general rule of thumb is to start with 12-point type and add a point for every decade after age 40. For instance, if a printed piece were to be targeted toward post-retirement individuals, appropriate type size would be 14 to 16 point (ages 50-79). As an individual's eyesight diminishes, it is easier to read larger type. This is another instance of where an accurately defined target audience can help in developing an appropriate printed piece.

- *Use only one or two different fonts within a single piece.* Although it may seem creative or fun to use more than two fonts, it tends to portray an amateur or childish appearance. When mixing two fonts together, it works best to mix a serif font (letters have ex-

Figure 11-2. Typical Type Point Sizes

12 point	14 point	16 point
18 point	24 point	

tensions or "feet" on the ends) with a sans serif font (letters do not have extensions on the ends) (see Figure 11-3).

- *Use CAPS, **bold**, or italics only to emphasize a word or main idea.* These tools are used to enhance a point. If they are used for more than a few words at a time, it becomes difficult to read and distinguish important ideas. Do not capitalize complete sentences or paragraphs. Full capitalization is hard to read and portrays a message of "shouting" (see Table 11-2).

- *Stick to simple fonts.* Fancy or script fonts are difficult for most readers and should be used sparingly. Script fonts are appropriate when trying to portray softness, sensitivity, or elegance. Be sure to use a large enough type when using script.

- *Serif versus sans serif.* Typically, serif type is easier to read than sans serif type (although sans serif is good for most headings). Sans serif is appropriate to use when trying to convey a sense of formality or professionalism. Due to the block lettering associated with sans serif type, it is also easier for individuals with failing eyesight to read. In contrast, serif is less formal and conveys a "softer" message (see Figure 11-3).

Graphics

Graphics take the monotony out of large volumes of text. Many can remember the disappointment they experienced when they read their first book without pictures. Chances are that the first "picture-free" book was read sometime around the sixth grade. Although most readers prefer illustrations, people with low-literacy or children may rely on them for guidance through text. Additionally, children and low-literacy readers are more likely to retain knowledge from graphical images, whereas more cognitive learners do fine with text. Using graphics can even help readers retain information for longer periods of time. Applying the following concepts to the use of graphics will ensure that they aid the reader.

- *Use graphics that precisely portray the message.* Graphics should aid the reader in comprehending and following the message. Individuals who have a difficult time comprehending a message tend

Figure 11-3. Serif and Sans Serif Type

SERIF (with feet)   **SANS SERIF** (without feet)

Table 11-2. Inappropriate Use of Capitalization

THIS IS AN EXAMPLE OF USING ALL UPPER CASE LETTERS. WHICH DO YOU
THINK IS EASIER TO READ, THIS PARAGRAPH OR THE ONE IMMEDIATELY
FOLLOWING?

This is an example of using a mixture of upper and lower case letters. Which do
you think is easier to read, this paragraph or the one immediately preceding it?

---

to use graphics as a guide. Therefore, a graphic should be placed
near the text that illustrate the idea. Do not include an inappropriate graphic just for the sake of having one. For example, do
not use pictures that are outdated (e.g., individual wearing wide
lapels). The reader may believe that the information is just as
outdated as the graphic.

- *Use simple line drawings as opposed to complex graphics.* Simple line
  drawings do not contain large amounts of detail and are easily
  recognizable. Complex graphics generally contain shading and
  intricate detail. As such, complex graphics may not be understood by the reader or may lose their clarity during reproduc-
  tion.

- *Use graphics that are appropriate for the target audience.* If the material is intended for the "general" public, graphics should represent cultural diversity and depict *positive* health behaviors. In
  general, pictures of people have more impact than pictures of
  objects. Ideally, a person should be shown acting out the positive health behavior being described. Also, pictures of women
  tend to portray more trustworthy than those of men. It is important, however, to avoid stereotyping or making assumptions
  about people or behaviors (e.g., not every family is made up of
  two parents, a boy, a girl, and a family dog with the mother as
  the primary caretaker).

- *Leave ample white space around graphics.* As with type, use a lot of
  white space around graphics. This will help the graphics draw
  the eye into the type rather than vice-versa. Also, avoid wrap-
  ping text around graphics as this is often hard to read.

- *Use varying sizes of graphical elements.* If graphics are all the same
  size, they are not very interesting. Instead, varying element sizes
  adds interest and shows what is most important. Size should
  depict the relative importance of each image.

- *Anchor graphics to the edge of the page.* Graphics should not be floating in the middle of the page. Instead, try to anchor them to the edge of the page to help balance the graphics with the text.

- *Use shading with caution.* Gray shading adds contrast when it is not possible to print in color. Shading, however, should never exceed 20% gray unless printing in reverse. Reverse means using white text on an all black background and should always be a 100% black background. This method should be used sparingly, and only to highlight an idea.

Readability

In public health, most materials must be developed for readers with low-literacy. It is estimated that the average person reads at a sixth-grade reading level. To be safe, many public health agencies write educational materials at a fourth-grade level. Even readers that have completed high school are probably not reading at a twelfth-grade level. Therefore, when developing materials for the general public, it is best to aim for a fourth- to sixth-grade reading level. This increases the likelihood that most readers will be able to comprehend the message.

There are a number of readability tests available that determine reading level. Many word-processing programs have built-in readability tests. Most readability formulas (e.g., SMOG, FOG, and FRY) are based on a system that compares the number of sentences in relation to the number of multisyllabic words within a passage. Materials that contain several short sentences consisting of short words will score at the lowest reading level. Many health educators, especially those just out of college, are accustomed to writing at a post-secondary level. It takes hard work and creativity to learn how to create materials that are interesting, simple, and accurate. Table 11-3 contains examples of how simple substitutions can be used for more difficult words.

Materials should be developed at the reading level at which they are intended to be used. They should not be written at a high reading level then lowered word-for-word. This method generally tends to lose part of

Table 11-3. Substituting Simple Phrases to Increase Ease of Reading

Word	Substitute
Carcinogens	cause cancer
Hypertension	high blood pressure
Accumulate	add up
Automobile	car

the intended message. If possible, the product should be developed in the same language in which it is to be used. Translation is never direct and meanings may get lost during the translation process. It is true that "literal, word-for-word translations may be offensive, incomprehensible, or culturally irrelevant."[2]

In addition to making sure that information is written at an appropriate reading level, a number of other points will ensure appropriate readability:

- *Caution using slang words.* Slang should be used with caution as it is not always appropriate and may offend some people. On the other hand, it is useful to use terms with which the target audience is familiar and to which they can relate.

- *Use of technical jargon.* Many people do not understand technical words, especially medical terms. For example, many readers confuse the meanings of words like "edema" and "enema." Obviously, this could seriously change the interpretation of the message. Keep it clear and simple. Sometimes it may be necessary to use difficult medical terms. For instance, a mammogram is a mammogram. Anytime a complicated term must be included, it should be defined or explained. A mammogram might be described as an x-ray of the breast tissue.

- *Active versus passive.* Use active rather than passive phrases (see Table 11-4). Vivid and active phrases make it clear to the reader exactly what is expected of them and what action to take.

- *Power words.* These are words that have been used for years by advertisers to elicit action from the reader. Although these words are most often used in product marketing, they can be used by health educators to guide the reader into action. They usually are included in headlines (see Table 11-5).

TYPES OF PRINTED MATERIALS

Printed materials come in a wide array of formats serving a variety of purposes. Target audience, purpose, and length all play a role in determining which format will best suit the information being presented. The creator may have the freedom to choose which to use. In general, health educators use four basic types of printed materials to communicate their message: Newsletters, pamphlets, flyers, and posters/billboards. In addition to the basics, there are other formats in which to distribute information that will be briefly discussed at the end of this section.

Table 11-4. Active Versus Passive Phrases

ACTIVE:	Eat five servings of fruits and vegetables every day.
PASSIVE:	For better health, five servings of fruits and vegetables should be eaten every day.
ACTIVE:	Exercise three times a week for good health.
PASSIVE:	Getting regular exercise promotes good health.

Newsletters

Newsletters are used to communicate information and educate large numbers of readers at regular intervals. They are typically used for (1) communicating specific information to a particular group on a regular basis (e.g., quarterly updates to coalition members), (2) raising awareness (e.g., HIV / AIDS issues in the community to registered voters), (3) promoting services (e.g., health department services and events to school personnel), and (4) raising money (e.g., charitable organization updates to past contributors). It is important to know the exact purpose prior to initiating development of a newsletter so that the basic layout can be tailored to the designated purpose. It can be challenging to plan a newsletter because varying (and unknown) amounts of information needs to be placed into a relatively stable format. The amount of information is likely to fluctuate from one issue to the next.

Many decisions need to be made when developing a newsletter, including the following:

- *Who is the target audience?* The target audience for the newsletter will dictate the information that it contains, the reading level, the layout, artwork, title, and much more. It is very important to know exactly who the audience is and to keep them in mind during all stages of development. Knowing how to cater to the target audience will make it easier to capture their interest. For example, past contributors to a charitable organization are probably interested in knowing where their contribution is going and that it is going to a good cause.

- *What is the purpose of the newsletter?* Newsletters are developed and distributed for a variety of reasons. They can be used for promoting services, providing updates to a membership or group, education, and networking.

- *How much information should the newsletter include?* Certain elements often appear in every newsletter. These may include cal-

Table 11-5. Power Words

Free	Introducing	Improved	Proven
Offer	It's Here	How-to	You
New	Announcing	The Truth About	Why
Amazing	At Last	Quick	Wanted
Startling	Easy	Sensational	Quick
Magic	Results	Suddenly	Last Chance

endars, personal interviews, feature articles, updates, letters to the editor, a table of contents, or contests and quizzes. Essentially, a newsletter is a miniature newspaper. During the initial planning of the newsletter, sections should be determined.

It is much easier to plan for extra space than trying to fit too much information into too little space. A rule of thumb is to plan for 20% more space than what is originally predicted to be needed. It is better to have extra white space than to have text crammed together. The final number of pages needs to also be taken into account. Most newsletters are made up of an even number of pages (2,4,6,8) to best utilize space and to be cost effective. If the newsletter is to be stapled, the number of pages should be divisible by four (4,8,12). Printers may add extra charges for stapling a newsletter and inserting loose pages.

- *How will the newsletter be laid out?* Newsletters leave plenty of room for individual creativity by the developer, but should consist of a basic underlying "grid" format. Because newsletters are generally re-created weekly, monthly, quarterly or even annually, effective planning before the first edition is crucial for consistency and ease. Creating a basic grid format will assist developing the components and layout of a newsletter.

   Newsletters can be rather dull if they contain too much text with too few graphical elements. A way of checking layout is to place a dollar bill horizontally at the top of each page and run it down the page. The dollar bill should be touching at least one graphical element at all times. If not, the reader will probably lose interest.

- *How will the newsletter be distributed?* A plan for distribution should be determined during the initial planning phase. If it is to be mailed, will it be a self-mailer or stuffed into an envelope? If it is to be a self-mailer, space should be planned on the back page for mailing labels and postage. If it is to be stuffed into an envelope, the size of the newsletter or envelop needs to be taken into consideration. Determining these ahead of time will aid in planning an accurate budget. If the newsletter is to be displayed in a rack, the heading (masthead) is crucial to grab the reader's attention.

- *How often will the newsletter be developed?* Time, cost, and quantity of information are the factors that will determine the schedule of development and distribution. How much information needs to be distributed? Can it be done annually or quarterly? If there is an abundance of information, it may be necessary to develop it weekly or monthly. Also, how important is it that information be timely in order to be useful? For example, if the newsletter is to be used to promote services, a monthly newsletter would probably be more useful than an annual one.

- *How can information be presented in an interesting fashion?* The more interactive a newsletter is, the more readers are likely to read it. The following make a newsletter more interesting for the reader: (1) Hold a contest for a newsletter title to create ownership for the target audience, (2) pull interesting quotes from articles and enlarge them to grab the readers attention (this will pass the dollar bill test), (3) use drawings by children as artwork, or (4) provide something interactive, such as a crossword, quiz, or a recipe.

Pamphlets

Pamphlets are one of the most basic methods for disseminating health education information. Pamphlets may supplement presented material, supply information at health fairs, be mailed to a group of people with a common health problem or interest, or act as resource materials in waiting rooms, schools, and doctor's offices. If not designed effectively, however, they can be a waste of time, money, and resources. People generally take about seven seconds to decide if they want to open the pamphlet and read further. Therefore, it is important that the cover grab the reader's attention and invite them to continue reading. If the individual does not believe that the information is personally pertinent, the material will not be read. For example, consider a diabetes pamphlet in a hospital waiting room. If the pamphlet is designed for the "general population" and has a picture of a young Caucasian woman on the cover, who is most likely to pick up the material to read it? Probably not a middle-aged, African-American male. The cover should accurately convey that the information is for either one specific group or the general population. There are four cover elements that can be used to gain the target audiences attention: (1) Effective graphics, (2) a catchy title, (3) supplemental information (e.g., subtitles, summary statement), and (4) following a "Z" pattern.

Many individuals believe that a pamphlet can be developed in a short amount of time by sitting in front of a computer and combining words with pictures. Pamphlet development is a *process*. More than one person needs to be involved in this process. Ideally, the intended audience should be involved in the planning, development, and evaluation of the piece. If possible, a pamphlet should be field tested prior to wide distribution. This is especially important if the material undergoes translation.

Pamphlets are limited in space and, therefore, should contain only "need to know" information rather than "nice to know" information. "Need to know" information is that which the reader *needs* in order to understand and assimilate the main point of the message. The pamphlet should begin and end with the primary message, and repeat the most important point(s) three times.

A list of local resources or avenues for the reader to obtain additional information should also be included. It is important to call any listed agencies *prior* to printing to make sure that they are in operation and can supply the information that is being claimed. Adding the date of development makes it easier to determine if the pamphlet is up-to-date, or if it needs to be revised.

Finally, pamphlets that are a part of a series, should all be planned at the same time. There will obviously be components that vary from one pamphlet to the next, but many of the elements should be the same (e.g., logo, artwork, format). This continuity will aid the reader in recognizing the pamphlet as a part of a series. If one pamphlet is effective, readers will be more likely to pick up another pamphlet that they recognize as a part of the same series.

Flyers and Posters

Flyers and posters seem relatively easy to develop because they are limited to one page. This can pose a challenge not encountered by lengthier printed educational materials—limited space and a large quantity of competition. Generally, flyers and posters only have a few seconds to attract the attention of the reader. Therefore the headline, or main message, must be clearly visible from some distance. Often, flyers and posters rely heavily on graphics and a strong message. It is important that all of the important information be included—who, what, where, how, and when.

Flyers

Flyers are relatively inexpensive to develop. Usually they are intended to be used to promote onetime events, activities, or services. Most flyers are printed on 8.5 x 11-inch paper. Because they must be seen from a distance, it is vital that the headline be large and legible. The headline should also attract the interest of the intended viewer so that they are motivated to come closer for additional information. Flyers rely heavily on graphics to help differentiate them from all of the other flyers in circulation. With any one-page printed material, the most important thing to keep in mind is that there is only one chance to make a first impression.

Flyers may be posted in hallways, on kiosks or on bulletin boards, or distributed by hand to individuals. Because of large-scale printing, it is not usually worthwhile to print in color. Instead, colored paper may be used to attract attention.

Posters

The same basics that apply to flyers also apply to posters. The main difference is that posters are intended to last longer. They may be more expensive due to the larger size and use of color. Billboards are essentially very large posters, that are expected to reach very large numbers of people. Billboards can be very costly, so it is essential to know the target audience.

Other Printed Materials

There are truly no limitations as to where information can be printed. Target audience research, or needs assessments, help determine which print format will work the best. Everyone is accustomed to seeing newsletters and pamphlets, but not everyone has received an educational message printed on bookmarks, calendars, restaurant place mats, or stickers. The important questions to keep in mind are who, where, when, and how will the information be received. If a health message is to be distributed by mail to members of a book club, why not send it printed on a bookmark? It is good to be creative and willing to take risks!

CONCLUSION

By following a systematic planning, development, and evaluation process for printed educational materials, health educators will assure that their message is communicated in a clear and meaningful way. Although every reader comes from a different social and educational background, all readers appreciate well-developed materials. Health educators often times have the freedom to choose which print format is most appropriate for the message that they intend to deliver. The creator of any successful piece must consider effective layout, fonts, graphics, and appropriate reading level. A good mix of these elements leads to a printed material that will have a positive impact on health behavior.

References

1. Timmerick, T. (1995). *Planning, program development, and evaluation.* Sudbury, MA: Jones and Bartlett.

2. Sabogal, F., Otero-Sabogal, R., Pasick, R., Jenkins, C., & Perez-Stable, E. (1996). Printed health education materials for diverse communities: Suggestions learned from the field. *Health Education Quarterly, 23*(supplement).

3. Siebert, L. , & Ballard, L. (1992). A good layout is. . ., *Making a Good Layout* (pp. 1-9). North Light Books.

Chapter 12

GRANT WRITING

Susan B. Dusseau, M.A., C.H.E.S.

Author's Comments: *No one I know started out to be a grant writer. From an administrative perspective, however, grant writing has become a necessity to agencies, as external funding is often needed in order to expand or improve existing programs. Although we often hear that grant dollars are scarce, this is not really the case. There are more sources for money than most people realize.*

Every health educator should have the opportunity to participate in seeking external funds. Through external funding, our agency has been able to help women save their lives through early detection of cancer. We have helped people finally break their addiction to nicotine, resulting in a significant improvement in their quality of life. It is gratifying to know that a program you created, for which you obtained external funding, can so positively impact entire families.

I began writing proposals within several years of starting my first full-time health education position. It took practice to feel confident at grant writing. I recommend that anyone interested in mastering grant writing should take advantage of continuing education opportunities associated with the process. How long it takes to master this skill depends on writing abilities and how frequently grant writing opportunities are pursued. Even if your job does not require writing grants, volunteer for a group where you can be on a committee that is responsible for seeking funds. It is a valuable experience, and you will find that there is tremendous satisfaction in leveraging resources for a worthy cause.

INTRODUCTION

As federal, state, and local governments seek to balance budgets and give relief to taxpayers, they are challenged to cut costs in expensive human welfare programs. These actions will increasingly impact programs at the local agency level where most human services are delivered. With a growing share of the nation's assets being funneled to curative health care costs, less dollars exist for prevention and health promotion programs. Programs, therefore, must compete for limited dollars and continuously seek out new sources of funding. Identifying funding sources and skillful grant writing are becoming essential for continued funding of community health education programs.

Many health education positions are funded through time-limited grants, especially for health educators working in nongovernmental agencies. Therefore, an individual's continued employment may rest on the ability to convincingly secure financial support. The ability to seek out and write grant proposals for sustaining and expanding programs is quickly becoming a priority job responsibility.

Fortunately, as the number of nonprofit organizations seeking outside funding continues to grow, the number of foundation and corporate funding sources has also been increasing. Conservative estimates indicate that over 500,000 agencies receive $50 billion each year.[1] Even though funding sources are available, the critical factor in whether or not a proposal is funded is related to how persuasively it is written. Only 1 in 10 proposals submitted, however, is actually funded.[1]

This chapter presents an overview of procedures and practical steps essential for effective grant writing, tips and techniques for success, and how to overcome barriers that impede grant funding. In order to better understand the discussion, the following terms are defined for the reader. *Grant writing* is the process of writing a proposal in order to obtain funding in the form of a grant. A *grant proposal*, is a "positive statement that sets forth an activity or program in such a way that its chances of being accepted [for funding] are maximized."[2] A *grant* is "the sum of money comprising an award of financial assistance to recipient individuals or organizations."[2]

PLANNING FOR GRANT PROPOSAL WRITING

Developing Partnerships

Organizations, both profit and nonprofit alike, are currently faced with streamlining in order to be as cost effective and productive as possible. One means of reducing costs, while remaining effective, is to collaborate, or partner, with organizations that are pursuing similar goals. These partnerships consist of two or more groups working together on programs designed to meet human needs, or prevent unnecessary problems. Collaborative efforts should be well-defined and mutually beneficial to all parties involved.

A collaborative approach increases the likelihood of success. For example, a local cancer agency may identify that single mothers with a child having cancer often need more ongoing help than is currently available. Meanwhile, a visiting nurse association may be in need of a better system to monitor children whose treatment team is two hours away. Working together could foster development of a plan that is more community focused, and incorporates groups that work directly with the target population. A more comprehensive service could be offered, and interagency communication could be enhanced. Multiplied experience and brain power, coupled with a greater likelihood of being funded, can benefit all agencies and clients involved.

Collaborative grant writing efforts also should occur within agencies. If the lead person in a grant writing process solicits internal input, a team can be formed to assist in the grant preparation. A supervisor with a track record of successful grant writing, a team of health educators, and a student intern, can be assembled so each has a specific role. For example, the Avon Corporation funds breast cancer awareness outreach projects twice per year. A local cancer agency administrator, an agency health educator, and a health education intern, could each write a section of the proposal, preventing the whole responsibility from falling on a single person. A combined effort of talents, experiences, and skills most likely will result in a more concise, yet thorough proposal.

Establishing a Strategic Plan

Strategic, or long-range, planning is the process by which organizational goals, objectives, and action plans are established. The process results in a sound, written document that should excite, convince, and motivate those who support the organization, especially funders. Strategic planning should be an integral part of every agency prior to pursuing external funding. An updated mission statement for the agency will be vital to developing the strategic plan, as it will be instrumental in determining grant writing direction. The agency's most recent planning document must also be readily available, so that as a proposal is prepared, it can clearly be shown that the program to be funded is a key part of the agency's overall mission. Additionally, the agency evaluation system or quality assurance program can be consulted and reviewed to retrieve data to be included within the grant proposal.

Assessing agency strengths and weaknesses can also aid in the development of the strategic plan. Identifying key agency characteristics will help to capitalize on agency strengths and minimize weaknesses. Relating how the agency strengths meet demonstrated community needs will best sell the program.

Strategic planning for grant writing includes (1) getting appropriate people together to discuss program and funding issues, (2) gathering resources and information to support a plan of action, (3) preparing a plan, (4) evaluating the progress, and (5) building on success. For example, effective planning associated with writing a grant to expand nutrition education services could include (1) discussing the idea with key agency staff and board members; (2) contacting other coordinators of nutrition oriented services such as a hospital dietitian, local extension home economist, or Women and Infant Children (WIC) program coordinator; (3) accessing a local library or the Internet to research information about the topic; (4) contacting other agencies in the community that have received a similar grant and asking if they would be willing to share a copy of their proposal; and (5) preparing a draft proposal and asking local professionals to provide feedback.

Locating Funding Sources

A critical component of proposal planning is the process of determining funding sources that will most likely support the program proposal. Once a list of potential funders is formulated, the most appropriate sources need to be identified. The most likely sources for funding are foundations and government contracts.

Foundation Funding

Foundations are private family, corporate, or community organizations with significant funds invested for the purpose of helping charitable agencies or educational institutions. Because local foundations usually award funds to organizations within their communities or nearby regions, pursuing this type of funding is often the best place to start. Many corporations, however, may be interested in funding programs outside of their area, if a likelihood of program replicability exists.

Foundation cycles are usually quarterly, biannual, tri-annual, or annual. Their purpose is to support as many worthwhile initiatives as possible with the funds they have available. Due to the number of requests and finite funding, smaller projects have a greater likelihood of being funded. In fact, 80% of foundation grants are for amounts under $5000.[1]

Many sources exist for locating foundations that fund health projects. Most public libraries have foundation directories available. The directors of local community foundations, a local agency such as the United Way, and grant writers employed by hospitals, universities, or other community agencies, can also assist in identifying funding possibilities. The Foundation Center, which publishes *The Foundation Directory*, is considered by many to be the best resource in the nation for information pertaining to foundations. This nonprofit corporation maintains reference collections at designated locations, usually in large cities, in every state. Other resources, such as *Getting a Grant in the 1990s: How to Write Successful Grant Proposals* by Robert Lefferts, include comprehensive lists of foundation directories and sources.[2] A librarian can be consulted for more information about funding sources. In addition, many foundation funding directories are available on the Internet (see Table 12-1 for Internet funding sources).

Table 12-1. Internet Funding Sources

Federal	
Catalog of Federal Dom. Asst.	http://www.gsa.gov:80/fdac/
GrantsWeb	http://web.fie.com/cws/sra/resource.htm
FedWorld	http://www.fedworld.gov/
USDHHS	http://www.os.dhhs.gov
SAMHSA	http://www.samhsa.gov/grant/gfa_kda.htm
NIH	http://www.nih.gov
CDC	http://www.cdc.gov/funding.htm
Foundations	
Council on Foundations	http://www.cof.org
The Foundation Center	http://fndcenter.org
Foundation sites	http://www.wmich.edu/research/funding.html

Government Funding

The *Catalog of Federal Domestic Assistance*, which can be ordered through the U.S. Government Superintendent of Documents or accessed via the Internet (http://www.gsa.gov:80/fdac/), is an excellent source for information pertaining to federal funding. Grant writers should be aware, however, that this document is quickly outdated. A computer-based program of the Catalog and a list of access points serving specific communities, is available from the U.S. General Services Administration. Local agencies should realize that federal funding is very tight and competitive, and usually difficult to receive unless a major collaboration exists among community agencies.

A variety of sources for governmental funding also exist at the state level. In Michigan, for example, funds are available from the Governor's Discretionary Fund, and Prevention Network mini-grants. The Governor's Discretionary Fund is directly controlled by an appointee of the Governor with dollars earmarked specifically for substance abuse prevention programs targeting adolescents. The Prevention Network mini-grant program is funded by the State Department of Community Health for substance abuse services. Nongovernmental associations (e.g., American Hospital Association) may have funding also, as might local sources, including civic groups (e.g., Rotary Club, Kiwanis Club, and Junior League).

A number of sources, such as disease-specific associations (e.g., American Cancer Society, American Heart Association), pharmaceutical companies, and the federal government, give priority to funding *research* proposals. These types of proposals, however, are usually research intensive and primarily written at the university level. Most community-based agencies focus on programs, rather than basic research, and therefore, will usually not vie for research proposals.

Gathering Information

Once potential funding sources have been identified, supportive data must be collected. A recent community needs assessment and improvement document (see Chapter 1, "Community Health Assessment and Improvement"), commissioned by the local health department or other community health agencies, will provide a summary of the current problems (e.g., substance abuse, violence) or priorities (e.g., services to people who lack health insurance) in the community. This information will be useful in determining the focus of the grant proposal. Other local agencies, such as the United Way or a community mental health agency, often have compiled similar data. Community planners, city council members, or county commissioners can also be contacted to determine what data or resources would provide insight on the most pressing local issues. Additionally, the agency should survey potential funders to determine which types of programs have been funded in recent years in the community. This will assist in determining which health issues will receive priority in funding.

Identifying Funding Source Requirements

A meeting between the funding agency representative and an organization spokesperson should be arranged, if possible, prior to grant proposal submission. This meeting will enable the organization to properly prepare the proposal according to funding guidelines. At this meeting, funding priorities and the process for submitting a proposal should be discussed. The organization representative should be prepared with a written project concept or outline (i.e., pre-proposal) consisting of a brief agency history, a description of previous funding efforts, the mission of the organization, a needs statement, and a summary of the proposed program. If a meeting is not possible, the funding agency representative should be asked the following questions:

- Is the funding agency interested in funding this type of project?
- How should a proposal be submitted?
- Is there an application form?
- When should the proposal be submitted?
- Is there any other information that will aid in the proposal process?

Following initial contact, some funding agencies will agree to preview a proposal before it is formally submitted. This preview can be arranged by a telephone call or letter. If possible, previously funded proposals should be reviewed to discover which topics are most likely to be funded.

An annual report, a list of the previous year's grantees, and a description of present areas of funding interest, can also provide valuable insight into the funder's priorities.

Funders should be informed if money will be requested from multiple sources. The organization must determine if the funding agency has previously granted partial or matching funding to be consistent with the funder's policy. Often, a plan for raising matching funds from another source is a desirable feature for attracting funders.

Funders will also want to know if the proposal is intended to support a new initiative (i.e., a pilot program), or to maintain regular program operating expenses. New initiatives are more likely to be funded. In many cases, however, "repackaging" a program or showing how it is evolving, conveys that it can now better meet evolving human needs. For example, in a Michigan community, a smoking cessation program was developed for low income residents as a result of a large pharmaceutical company donating nicotine patches. The supply of patches, however, was exhausted within five months and the program was discontinued. A second collaborative effort between the state and local health departments, a local cancer agency, and a different pharmaceutical company allowed the program to be reinstated. Program modifications were instituted and an improvement in client success rates was achieved with the "repackaged" program format.

Regardless of funding source, a relationship should be developed with the funding agency. The more a relationship is built with a funder, the more an agency will be perceived as a team player in the philanthropic arena. This relationship begins with the initial pre-proposal inquiry. Experts have suggested that chances for being funded increase by 300% if a pre-proposal contact is made with the funder.[3]

Determining Proposal Type and Format

Proposal Types
In general, six types of proposals exist: Program, research, training, planning, technical assistance, and capital improvement.

- *Program proposals* provide specific services. The majority of proposals written by community health practitioners will be program proposals. For example, a local substance abuse prevention agency facilitating interagency cooperation to reduce alcohol, tobacco and other drug problems, provides a specific community service.

- *Research proposals* study a health issue. For instance, a state college school of nursing could receive multiyear funding to survey the extent of problems associated with being a primary care giver for a person with a chronic illness. The results from the study would provide important input for the medical care system in better meeting the needs of families facing this health concern.

- *Training proposals* provide funding for "training-of-the-trainers" programs. An example would be funds being available from the State Chamber of Commerce Foundation to help local business representatives, in partnership with their local Chamber of Commerce, become trained to implement *Drugs Don't Work* programs in communities.

- *Planning proposals* provide planning, coordination, and networking for problem solving. For example, the first phase of the ASSIST grants, funded by the National Cancer Institute to reduce national smoking rates, was specifically instituted for planning purposes. Later phases, however, funded a variety of program initiatives, such as networking, to enact more restrictive policies on smoking. Health educators need to be aware that this type of proposal will not be the most likely to receive funding, as the social impact will occur long after programs are developed and successfully implemented.

- *Technical assistance proposals* assist other agencies with programs. For example, intermediate school district agencies often write grants designed to assist local districts with school and curriculum improvement projects.

- *Capital improvement proposals* are designed to acquire equipment, or construct or remodel a building. Community foundations are the most likely to fund tangible assets. Many nonprofit agencies, for example, have upgraded office systems as a result of community foundations responding to justified local needs.

Regardless of proposal type, the present and future human needs addressed by the program must be communicated to the funder. Agency uniqueness beyond the mission statement must be conveyed, along with how the organization is positioning itself over the next five years to serve people in the community. The proposal will ultimately be sold by capturing the essence of what the program does to benefit the community. For example, one cancer agency tripled the number of client encounters over a 10-year period while maintaining the same staffing levels. Significant growth in services was demonstrated, while maintaining expenses in a cost efficient manner. Client satisfaction surveys disclosed favorable ratings.

As a result of the community benefits indicated, a $25,000 capital improvement grant to upgrade workstations was awarded to the cancer agency.

Proposal Format

Depending on the funding source, proposal formats may vary. Formats may range from a one-page letter to a 20- or more page proposal. Proposal format examples include requests for proposals, contracts with state agencies, four-page concept papers, and pre-proposals.

Request For Proposals (RFP) are usually solicited opportunities from governmental agencies to design and implement programs. An agency that has received governmental funding in the past will probably be on the mailing list to receive RFPs as they become available. If not, governmental agencies should be contacted to ensure future announcements are sent to the agency. Applicants are provided with detailed instructions for completing the RFP. Instructions generally include guidelines, proposal format and evaluation criteria, budget forms and preparation instructions, and attachments. The proposal that is developed as a response to an RFP must be submitted by a specific deadline. Additionally, the funder's advice should be sought while writing the proposal, as this will provide insight into funder criteria and requirements for proposal submission.

Contracts with state agencies are often similar in format to RFPs. They tend to have longer narrative sections describing the details of the project and have more comprehensive budget and activity reporting requirements.

A *four-page concept paper* is a condensed version of the project and rarely includes extras such as letters of support. Usually, a simple budget, rather than a detailed budget and budget narrative, is all that is necessary.

A *pre-proposal* is often in the form of a letter or a simple two-page explanation. It describes a community need, the proposed plan to meet the need, proposed cost, and why the soliciting agency is in the best position to make an impact.

COMPONENTS OF A GRANT PROPOSAL

Proposals can have varying components depending on the size of the program and funder requirements. For example, foundations often use a standard application requiring less extensive financial detail, while government RFPs typically require multiple sections of cost and budget explanation. Basic proposal components usually include the following:

1. Cover letter or summary

2. Introduction

3. Problem or needs statement

4. Objectives

5. Methods of Implementation

6. Evaluation strategies

7. Plans for continued funding

8. Budget

9. Supplementary materials

Cover Letter or Summary

The cover letter, or summary, condenses the total proposal into a concise, one-page request. It should be written to the funding executive's attention on agency letterhead. The cover letter is constructed after completing the proposal in order to highlight main features from each section. A table of contents is often included with a lengthy proposal, but is not necessary for most concise program proposals.

Introduction

The introduction of the grant proposal should include agency qualifications, a brief history of the organization, the organization's most noteworthy accomplishments, and other community agencies' support for the organization. Future plans of the organization, its demonstrated ability to conduct programs, and its mission statement should also be included.

Problem or Needs Statement

The problem or needs statement should describe the gap between what currently exists and what needs to be funded externally. To formulate a convincing rationale, grant writers could utilize (1) research findings, such as those reported from a local community agency or university; (2) survey data, often from random telephone interviews; (3) key informant interviews (e.g., target population leaders or experts); (4) focus group results, such as those conducted by medical centers to facilitate service expansion planning; (5) demographic information and statistics, which can be obtained from governmental planning entities; and (6) results of community assessment and improvement processes published by local health departments. Data collected at the local level regarding the target population will be more valuable than national statistics.

A grant writer should build a sense of urgency in the needs statement without over exaggerating. Many ideas can be conveyed, such as how the problem evolved in the community and how it will be minimized by the proposed program. The evaluation results of past programmatic efforts, and how the agency will respond to the need, must also be discussed. A problem statement needs to be written in terms of the RFP or granting agency objectives and criteria. The statement should focus on the importance of how this problem ties into the funder's mission.

Objectives

Program objectives should be measurable, time limited, outcome based, achievable, and relevant. The objectives state the process, outcomes, and roles of the health educators and target population. Action verbs such as "improve," "increase," "provide," "reduce," and "facilitate" should be used. As a general rule, the larger the project, the greater the number of corresponding objectives. Objectives serve as the basis for evaluating program efficiency and effectiveness.

Outcome objectives relate to the benefits achieved due to the success of the program. In contrast, process objectives refer to the completion of tasks over the course of the grant. An example of a process objective would be "to complete the recruitment of 150 eligible participants by the end of the first 60 days of the grant period." Process objectives are crucial for determining time lines, staff tasks, and whether plans need to be adjusted due to unforeseen events.

Methods of Implementation

Just as important as stating *what* will be done, is *how* it will be done. The methods section of the grant proposal describes the activities designed for achieving program objectives. It should be theory-based and show the uniqueness of the program. This information will provide support and be the basis for convincing funders why the proposal should be funded over other proposals submitted. A time line, or flowchart, (e.g., GANTT, PERT) should be constructed to show the series of action steps to be taken in the program. Listing activities on a time line will provide a clear way of showing program details. The necessary staffing, along with their program responsibilities, should also be described. Client descriptions may be included in this section. The methods section often is the most scrutinized, because this is where the uniqueness of the approach is described.

Evaluation Strategies

A comprehensive program evaluation consists of process, impact, and outcome evaluation components. An evaluation is necessary to show funders that the program achieved the stated objectives as planned. The types of data to be collected and how they will be analyzed and disseminated should also be included. Process evaluation determines the extent to which process objectives were met by examining how the implementation unfolded, and whether or not the original plan was followed. Employees and clients can complete surveys to help measure the process. Impact and outcome evaluation determine if outcome objectives for the program were met. Pretests and post-tests, for example, determine whether clients attained desired content. Program strengths and weaknesses, as well as ideas for improvement, can be determined from collected data.

Funding agencies will often outline what is expected for the evaluation section. If the proposal is a onetime request for equipment, evaluation may not be important. Large proposals, however, might warrant contracting with an outside evaluator from a university or private consulting firm. For most programs, community agencies will conduct their own evaluations.

A significant benefit of evaluation data is that it can be packaged into a powerful public relations tool for the agency. For example, news releases to local media, and summaries in newsletters to key supporters, can be developed. These may increase chances for future funding. In addition, when funders are weighing whether to support a future program proposed by the agency, a deciding factor may be that previous programs generated favorable community comment (e.g., letters to the editor).

Funding Continuation

Sustainability of the program will be important to funders after the grant period, typically 12-18 months, ends. Funders want to be part of the building process of a strong, meaningful program, but usually do not provide ongoing funds. In some situations, foundations may, for example, sponsor an annual lectureship in honor of a significant person, or support ongoing costs of an exceptional smaller program. Some programs will leverage a larger dollar value by the inherent structure, such as a program that purchases seed for low income people to plant gardens. With this local project, a foundation that specifically targets nutrition programs will find that their investment saves clients money, teaches a useful skill, and improves clients' health. Ideally, a permanent funding plan for the program is desirable. The agency may eventually be able to integrate the ongoing program costs, after the higher start-up costs have been met. Sometimes a plan to generate user fees is possible, or another funding source becomes available. For a program to survive, however, viable strategies for continuation funding and program sustainability will be essential.

Budget

The budget is a realistic projection of program costs. The dollars requested in the budget should match program activities. A budget form may be provided by the funder requesting expense information. RFPs, for example, always include the exact budget items necessary for implementation. If not requested, a listing of itemized expenses should be generated, including salaries, employee benefits, consultants fees, travel, supplies, equipment, rent, and other similar items. These comprise the direct costs, or the budget items that represent the direct expenditure of funds.[2] In contrast, indirect costs are items incurred by the grantee that are not readily identified as direct expenditures, but are necessary to facilitate and maintain operations for the programs.[2] These include such items as administrative overhead, building maintenance, and depreciation. Calculating indirect costs will depend on many variables, including the policy of the funder, and federal formulas. Table 12-2 includes a sample detailed budget request for $75,000.

Following direct and indirect expenses, a budget justification statement (i.e., how much money is being requested and why) should be included in narrative form. In-kind matches and other local funding should be explained in this section. A dollar amount (e.g., the projected cost for secretarial support) or a general description should be included for in-kind matches.

Supplementary Materials

Letter of Intent
Due to the large number of requests for support, funders may require a simple summary of the proposal. This summary may be called a letter of intent, letter of inquiry, pre-proposal letter, proposal letter, letter of interest, or prospectus. A letter of intent will enable preliminary screening by the funder, during which time suggestions may be made for program modification. Although a simple letter may suffice for a small monetary request (e.g., less than $10,000), requests for larger amounts will require more documentation elaborating on program need, strategies, and potential impact.

Appendices
Appendices are necessary for including supportive materials that would disrupt the flow of ideas if presented along within the text. These appear at the end of the grant proposal and include such items as (1) well-written letters of support from partner agencies, (2) a copy of the agency's annual report, (3) proof of nonprofit status, (4) a list of board members and key staff, (5) a balance sheet from the last annual audit, and (6) vitae of persons directly involved with the proposed program.

Each of the above items will enhance the program's appeal to a funding agency. For example, letters of support from partner agencies should be included with the submission of a sizable grant involving the cooperation of a number of agencies. Some funders place more value on letters of support than others. Also, inclusion of an agency annual report will support the viability of programs and services by providing an account of program and financial information. Nonprofit agency status can be demonstrated by inclusion of documents verifying this status. A letter with the agency's federal tax-exempt number may also be used as proof of nonprofit status. Additional appendices might include a list of board members and key staff that will lend credibility to the diverse representation and qualifications of the organization's central players. A balance sheet from the last annual audit can also be included to verify the income and expenses of the agency, and summarize fiscal health. The inclusion of vitae of the persons directly involved with the proposed program identify past grant, research, and programmatic experiences; further justifying their qualifications.

TIPS AND TECHNIQUES FOR SUCCESSFUL GRANT WRITING

Criteria for a Polished Proposal

A well-prepared grant proposal is best when it includes the funder's mission, yet is client driven. Throughout the proposal narrative, statements

Table 12-2. Sample Program Budget

Direct Expenses	
Personnel	
Salaries	
Program Supervisor- $40,000 @ .25 FTE	10,000
Health Educator- $26,000 @ 1.00 FTE	26,000
Secretary- $18,000 @ .30 FTE	5,400
Total Salaries	41,400
Fringe Benefits	
Calculated @ 25% of salaries of $41,400	10,350
Other Than Personnel	
Travel 5,000 miles @ .30	1,500
Supplies	2,690
Printing and Mailing	2,500
Total Other Than Personnel	6,690
Total Direct Expenses	58,440
Indirect Expenses	
Calculated @ 40% of salaries of $41,400	16,560
Total Expenses	$75,000

should reflect the benefits the target population will gain as a result of the program. An effective proposal should (1) have a calculated plan; (2) follow a logical and sequential flow from one idea to another; (3) use simple words, in brief sentences, and short paragraphs; (4) avoid jargon, acronyms, and generalizations; (5) minimize use of adjectives and adverbs; (6) balance the combination of statements, statistics, quotes, and case examples; (7) include useful charts and graphs; and (8) be written from the funder's point of view, clearly showing the benefits to the funder.

A calculated plan will show that each procedure in the proposed program was well thought out and sequential. Text should be easy to follow, using a tone that is clear, brief, and specific. Run-on sentences, and pompous words or phrases should be avoided. Illustrations, including statistics, case examples, and quotes, will support assumptions, as long as care is taken not to bore the reader with too many numbers. Pictures are often more beneficial than written narrative, so charts and graphs should be used when appropriate. Lastly, the funder's point of view must be considered at all times so the benefits of the proposal are understood.

Reporting Requirements

Most funders require communication about the program's progress during the funding cycle with quarterly and midyear reports being most frequently requested. A form will usually be provided by the funder to guide the grantee in adequately describing the program progress as compared to the original proposal. At the end of the program, a summary report should be sent to the funder with project results. Doing so will not only show agency initiative, but also the value of the relationship with the funder. This report will also alert the granting agency to any roadblocks during program implementation. Program implementation does not always happen as planned, and funders will want to know if targeted objectives were not met. Unanticipated benefits derived from the program can also be included in the summary report. If any progress reports will be delayed, the funder needs to be informed as soon as possible.

Thank You Notes

Regularly thanking the funder is an important part of all phases in the grant writing process. For example, a verbal thank you should follow a planning meeting, with a written note mailed once the proposal is sent. An appropriate method of recognition needs to be chosen for each individual who had some involvement in the project.

Thanking the funder can make a lasting impression, and is critical to effective relationships. The proposal cover letter should thank the funder for the potential opportunity to assist in bringing a needed program to the community. Peers from other community agencies and colleagues who provided consultation should also be thanked, whether or not funding is received. Collaborators appreciate knowing the proposal's funding status—a thank you note can easily be included with this information. Even participants in the program can be thanked with a token gift for their roles in helping the agency meet community needs.

Review Criteria

All grants are reviewed by an established committee of the funding organization or a group of pre-selected consultants. The committee's responsibility will be to objectively rate how the essential grant components convey a well-conceived and logical plan. The proposal has the best chance of obtaining a high score when written from the funders's perspective in a lively, informative, and concise manner. Figure 12-1 consists of a typical review criteria score sheet.

Time Lines

Keeping on track with activities is as important during the proposal development stage as during program implementation. When the grant proposal due date is set, a realistic sequencing of tasks and meetings helps everyone on the team be clear on expectations. These time lines may need to be modified as proposal activities progress.

STRATEGIES FOR OVERCOMING BARRIERS

Discouragement

The process of grant writing is tedious and can be discouraging at times. Initiating the process of writing a grant without consulting others can be a mistake, especially if inexperienced. Seasoned grant writers can provide the best advice for starting a proposal and will help troubleshoot when problem situations arise. Most will gladly review a proposal before it is sent to the funder. These individuals are often found in local health departments, intermediate school districts, universities, hospitals, and city or county planning departments. The director of a community foundation may be able to recommend local people with solid grant writing skills.

Due to administrators' and staff workers' schedules, it may be difficult to arrange times for planning team meetings. This difficulty should not be interpreted as a sign of disinterest or lack of cooperation, but as a challenge. Delegating tasks to planning team members will help in avoiding one person becoming overwhelmed, and will minimize feelings of discouragement.

Figure 12-1. Review Criteria

Available Points

Needs Assessment (15) _____

Project Objectives (15) _____

Project Design (10) _____

Formal Linkages/Collaborations (15) _____

Capacity of the Organization (10) _____

Project Staffing, Work Plan, & Time Lines (5) _____

Evaluation (10) _____

Budget (10) _____

Required Documents (10) _____

Total Score (100) _____

Lack of Appropriate Funding Sources

A situation could occur in which available funding sources will not be appropriate matches for a program. Wealthy individuals or businesses (e.g., banks) in the community are usually approachable for smaller funding needs (less than $10,000). Civic groups, such as the Rotary Club, Kiwanis Club, or Junior League, are examples of other community organizations committed to providing financial assistance, and perhaps even volunteers, for timely community projects. The local Chamber of Commerce, or a volunteer center, may be able to suggest which groups are receptive to grant proposals. Additionally, proceeds from a community event (e.g., a walk/run, a benefit concert) could be earmarked for a worthy project. A proposal letter to a civic organization asking for a commitment for such an event would be required.

Inadequate Communication

Communication may be a weak point either in the agency or with collaborating partners. Intentions for pursuing a grant should be announced at staff or departmental meetings. Also, key individuals from all involved agencies must be kept informed during the entire proposal process. Keeping a file or notebook of all planning documents, correspondence, and planning meeting minutes (with copies sent to committee members in a timely manner) ensures that the grant writing team and lead agency administration will be kept abreast of progress. A verbal thank you, personal notes, and small gifts are ways to reinforce continued participation and enthusiasm. Also, key people in the community should be kept informed of progress throughout the planning and implementation phases.

EXPECTED OUTCOMES

A grant writer must be prepared to receive feedback from the funder. Rejection or constructive criticism should not be taken personally, as learning occurs regardless of the outcome. Many times, rejection may have nothing to do with the quality of a proposal (e.g., the funder's allocation for the year has been spent, the focus of funding has changed, numerous quality proposals were submitted). In the case of rejection, reviewer comments should be requested and used for improvements.

Sometimes funders will negotiate specifics within the proposal. For example, the funder may offer a lesser dollar amount than what was requested. It must be determined if the program can be successfully implemented in a scaled-down format. If not possible, this should be stated to the funder in an honest, straightforward, and friendly manner. Reacting graciously may improve the chances of being funded in the future. Another reply from the funder may be a suggestion for an alternative plan. For example, the funder might request collaboration with another agency that has submitted a similar project. Being open to possible modifications of the original proposal by including other community agencies may increase chances of receiving funding.

The best possible feedback will be that the proposal has been funded. When this is the case, the good news should be shared in a timely fashion with everyone involved. News releases should be prepared to capitalize on the public relations front. Some length of time may have passed since submission of the grant proposal, so the grant time line should be rechecked, and meeting times arranged to keep the program on schedule. In most cases, the ownership of the materials developed as a result of the grant become the property of the agency submitting the grant (unless government funded). An expected courtesy, however, will be to acknowledge the funder in program materials. Upon receiving funding notice, the funders should be thanked for the grant. In addition, it is important to set aside time to celebrate the success. It will be much deserved!

CONCLUSION

Writing a grant proposal and having it funded will be an important milestone in the career of a health educator. Developing expertise in this area will make health educators even more important, as agencies continue to respond to growing community needs with little internal funding. Nurturing relationships with all segments of the community, coupled by confidence, will boost chances for future success in the fund-raising arena.

References

1. American Association of Fund Raising Councils. (1995). *Giving USA annual report.*

2. Lefferts, R. (1990). *Getting a grant in the 1990s: How to write successful grant proposals.* New York: Simon & Schuster.

3. Artley, D. P. (1997). Effective resource development for community based nonprofits and governmental agencies. Workshop proceedings, January 22-24, Okemos, MI.

Chapter 13

USING TECHNOLOGY

Robert J. Bensley, Ph.D.

Author's Comments: *Technology. Some love it. Some don't. Some see it as a tool to improve the way in which the world works, others see it as a force that will ultimately destroy the fabric of our society. Regardless of how you look at it, it is here, and it is now, and it is not going to go away. As a health educator who is trying to stay "on the bus" as we move into the world of high-speed computers and communication, I feel pretty fortunate. Having had the opportunity to study computer science as an undergraduate and then see the world from the eyes of "Big Blue" (a.k.a. IBM, which used to be big and used to be blue), I pretty much convinced myself that no matter what changes in technology took place, I could handle it. After all, Big Blue is Big Blue, isn't it? They set the stage for change, don't they? Needless-to-say, I was wrong. When it comes to the rapid technological advances that occur daily, I soon became aware that we are all along for the ride. It is enough just to hang on to the edge of the seat and hope that when you are tossed, the impact will not be too discomforting.*

Therefore, the purpose of this chapter: It is designed to assist local health educators, those who are already overburdened and spend their days on the front line, be aware of the technology currently available and how it can be used. Because of the enormity and complexity of technology, it would be nearly impossible (and absolutely boring) to present it in its entirety. Thus, I have attempted to take those bits and pieces that are most pertinent to health education and provide practical examples of how they can be used in our work. I encourage you to pick what you need from this chapter and apply it. Use it. Do something with it. But whatever you do, do not wait to "see what is going to happen" in the future. It's already here.

INTRODUCTION

Over the past 20 years, since the arrival of the world's first microcomputers, technology processes have been infused into the daily functioning of both the workplace and society. In only a short time, technology has evolved exponentially from the complex and cumbersome command-driven personal computers of the 1970s and 1980s (e.g., Apple IIe and IBM PC), through the incorporation of the graphic user interface (i.e., "point and click" technology), to the present day worldwide connections and access associated with the Internet. The technological revolution has become the catalyst for global interactions, economic growth, and the ever-increasing accumulation of information and knowledge.

The microprocessor has become an essential component in almost all advanced technological products and services. For instance, automobiles built in the 1970s and 1980s were comprised primarily of mechanical components. When a malfunction occurred, diagnosis consisted of merely testing a series of mechanical processes until the malfunctioning part or system was found. Automobiles today are still comprised of mechanical devices but are increasingly driven by complex microprocessor systems. Diagnosis no longer consists of listening for a "leaking hose" or a "clicking sound," but rather testing the car's systems with varied computerized diagnostic machines. Basically, microprocessors testing the functionality of other microprocessors. Virtually every mechanical device of yesteryear has been modified to include microprocessor technology.

Within the health education profession, technological advances have resulted in greater access to data, more complex research, and increased mechanisms for delivery of services. Health educators have become dependent on the technological expansions of the past two decades. Consider conducting a time series evaluation of the impact that a media campaign has on community attitudes and behaviors. Thirty years ago, the data analysis for this task would have been insurmountable. Through the use of computers and data analysis programs, the task today is relatively simple. Similarly, microcomputer applications allow health educators to develop, distribute, and track monthly newsletters without ever having to leave their desks. This task would have been an enormous undertaking as little as 10 years ago.

The above illustrations are only two of the many examples that depict the impact technology has had on the health education practitioner. This chapter is designed to assist practitioners understand the need for technology in the delivery of health education, avenues for incorporating technology into health education processes, and mechanisms for overcoming barriers.

THE NEED FOR TECHNOLOGY IN HEALTH EDUCATION

Technology in health education has been driven by the overwhelming need for finding more efficient and effective ways to assist populations in preventing or changing negative health behaviors. Even though methods for delivering health education messages and services continue to evolve, negative health practices still abound.

The need for technology in the delivery of health education is great. How technology can be used to address this need will be covered in the next section, 'Using Technology in Conducting Health Education Processes.' The use of technology is based on the need to:

- *Be more effective and efficient with less resources.* Like many other human service organizations, traditional health education agencies (e.g., health departments, hospitals, and community-based organizations) are in the midst of experiencing drastic budget reductions. Health educators are currently faced with providing services for a multitude of at-risk populations with only a fraction of the funding available from past years. It is not uncommon for a health education agency to have a single health educator taking on the responsibilities that two or three people would have shared in the past. At a time when terms such as downsizing are prevalent, health educators are often taxed with overwhelming pressures to provide comprehensive and effective services. Funding has become such a problem that many health educators must devote a large percentage of their limited time to the acquisition and management of external funding. Additional responsibilities, such as grant writing, coupled with the ever-increasing trend of depreciating agency funding, makes it nearly impossible for a health educator to function effectively without using current technologies. If not for computer technology, what would have been accomplished by two or three individuals 20-years ago would be nearly impossible by lone individuals today.

- *Provide more effective mechanisms for influencing the masses.* Delivery of health education services in the 1970s and 1980s consisted primarily of one-on-one or one-on-many approaches. Many of the health education approaches used during this period focused on education in the classroom and traditional mass media (e.g., television, radio, and newspaper). Although state-of-the-art for the era, these methods were limited in relation to efficiently reaching the masses needed to truly impact the problem. Current practices are now likely to include the induction of community-based coalitions, and media and legislative advocacy designed to empower the community to influence policy makers. Although these new methods provide additional approaches for reaching the general public, they are still limited to how efficiently and effectively they reach the masses.

- *Keep up with the rapid increase in new information.* The collective knowledge of all that is and has ever been known, is doubling every few years. Considering that it took thousands of years from the beginning of recorded history for knowledge to double the first time, doubling every few years is difficult to comprehend. With an increased database of available knowledge, a means of accessing that information needs to exist. Health educators can no longer depend on dated materials to provide them with up-to-date information, statistics, models, and approaches.

- *Access discussion groups and problem-solving forums.* As health educators take on more responsibilities with less resources, they have fewer colleagues with whom they can share ideas and seek feedback. Many health educators work in environments in which they are the only health educator on staff. In rural areas especially, many lone health educators are geographically separated from their colleagues. At least in an urban setting, health educators from individual agencies are able to interact at (e.g.) regular community coalition meetings. Without a mechanism for collective thought with other like professionals, health educators have a greater likelihood of being limited in the relation to providing quality, timely, and effective health education services.

- *Justify programs.* Being a non-income producing profession, the cost-benefit ratio of health education is constantly being scrutinized. In a world in which programming is dependent on external funding, it is vital that health educators are able to accurately measure program impact and communicate the need for allocated resources. Funding is dependent on being able to show the impact of health education programming. Therefore, complex and varied evaluation methods must be incorporated into program services. No longer can program efforts be reported by descriptive statistics alone. Health educators must be able to design and implement impactful evaluative studies of programming efforts. They must be able to accurately justify future programs based on their past and present successes.

- *Provide individuals with effective behavior change processes.* One of the major barriers that plagues health educators is the inability to directly impact the actions of individuals who engage in negative health behavior practices. Mass media and printed educational materials have provided a vehicle for communicating messages to the masses. Workshops and seminars have linked health educators with groups of individuals with specific health needs. Legislation has resulted in changes in policies and laws. Community coalitions have enabled communities to impact the culture and environment in which people live. Even so, efforts still fall short. Much of the failure associated with these approaches is due to the lack of ability to provide effective behavior change processes directly to those with the greatest need.

USING TECHNOLOGY IN HEALTH EDUCATION

Technology can be applied to health education in many ways. The complexity of using current technology can range from using a simple word processing program to create a letter, to broadcasting a seminar across the nation using satellite distance learning. The technology currently exists. It is a matter of getting health educators to understand how and when to access and utilize these available resources. Current technology applications that can be used to enhance the delivery of health education include (1) the Internet, (2) electronic mail, (3) personal assessment and behavior change applications, (4) desktop publishing and graphic art applications, (5) presentation software, (6) distance learning, (7) data analysis programs, and (8) program management applications.

The Internet

The Internet is an electronic network of computers connected to each other via traditional communication lines. Originally sponsored by the U.S. Department of Defense in the 1960s, the Internet has since become a worldwide avenue for sharing and accessing information.[1] It has made information that was once nearly impossible to attain available to anyone connected via a computer and modem. Within just a short period, the Internet evolved from a government defense project to an international vehicle, or "super highway," for accessing information. Millions currently use the Internet on a daily basis with forecasts that 300 million people worldwide will be connected by the year 2000.[1]

Central to the Internet is the World Wide Web (WWW or "web"), which provides an avenue for browsing and retrieving information. Introduced in 1994, the web provided the graphical user system that was missing from earlier Internet services such as Gopher, FTP, and Telnet.[2] The web is based on the concept of *hypertext*, which allows users to link from a document that is stored on one computer to a document that may be stored on another computer at a completely different site. It uses an addressing system known as Uniform Resource Locators (URLs) to locate the computer systems where documents actually exist. Within the URL (e.g., http://www.cdc.gov), the computer application protocol (http), Internet application (www), and actual address of the computer where the document resides (cdc.gov) are usually specified. Each site, or *page*, that is connected to the Internet has a unique URL. The start-up pages for each site are commonly referred to as "home pages."

Web browsers (e.g., Netscape Communicator, Microsoft Internet Explorer) are user-interface software packages that allow users to access the web. The browser becomes the access point from which an end user can search for sites and documents, create home pages, and retrieve data. Browsers allow the user to simply point and click rather than having to remember commands and URLs of specific sites.

One of the main advantages of browsers is the ability to access Internet search programs commonly referred to as *search engines*. In general, a search engine is an application that allows the user to search pre-designated indexes for specific keywords that are associated with specific web sites. In essence, search engines are automated index reviewers. Similar to thumbing through an index in the back of a book, a search engine thumbs through a web index looking for specified keywords.

A number of search engines already exist on the Internet (e.g., Yahoo, Lycos, Excite, Web Crawler, Infoseek). Therefore, the user does not need to purchase separate software in order to search the web. One question that may be raised is why so many different search engines exist. Is it really necessary to have multiple search engines? Because of the complexity and popularity of the web, no one search engine can keep up with the rapidly expanding Internet. Remember, search engines rely on an index of stored keywords. Even though engine indexes are constantly updated, it is nearly impossible to keep up with the new sites that are being added to the Internet on a daily basis. It has been estimated that the number of web sites doubles every 2 months.[3] Every search engine maintains its own index and searching approach. It is important to realize though, that search engines are likely to contain similar results. This is because search engines are only searching on indexes; they do not contain actual documents.

The way in which different search engines work can be related to shopping patterns at a grocery store. Some individuals shop by starting at the fruit and vegetable aisle located at the front of the store and wind up and down each aisle until they reach the last aisle. Others take just the opposite approach and begin at the far end of the store and work their way toward the front. Some rely on the signs located at the top of each aisle to find the categories of products for which they are searching. And still others sporadically move in and out of aisles until they have collected all the items on their list. Regardless of the method used, at the checkout line all consumers will have similar products in their carts. The brand and order may change, but the essence of the search is the same. So to with searching the web. Some search engines have a greater likelihood of accessing specific sites because of the keywords stored in their indexes. Regardless, the end result is fairly consistent.

Health educators can use the Internet for many purposes. In particular, the Internet provides health educators with the ability to (1) act as resource persons by creating and linking to sites containing educational or informational items, (2) access up-to-date information and state-of-the-art health education processes, and (3) link to grant funding agencies and foundations.

Act as Resource Persons

Many health education agencies and organizations have established web sites that pertain to their missions. Sites generally consist of information about the agency, dates of conferences and trainings, summaries of activities and events, findings from projects, content specific to the mission of the agency or organization, action-oriented materials (e.g., action alerts or press releases) and a mechanism for linking to other pertinent sites. A health education agency could create a home page and use it as a means for educating professionals about events and resources, educating the general public about issues, and providing links to other related sites. For instance, the contents of American Heart Association's home page (http://www.aha.org) includes information that pertains to the mission and activities of the association, current events, and press releases. In comparison, the American Cancer Society's home page (http://www.cancer.org) includes content related to prevention and treatment associated with different cancers and updates of current legislative issues. Many government agencies, such as CDC (http://www.cdc.gov), provide access to a multitude of research data, funding opportunities, weekly reports (e.g., *Morbidity and Mortality Weekly Report* at http://www.cdc.gov/epo/mmwr/mmwr.html), legislative issues, statistical trends, contact names, and the like. A number of sites also contain on-line searchable databases (e.g., the CDC *Wonder* database at http://wwwonder.cdc.gov), providing health educators with instant access to journal articles, statistical trends, and other pertinent information and data. Because of the immensity of the web, it is impossible to provide a comprehensive list of relevant web sites here. The reader is referred to *Web Sites for Health Professionals*, by Mark Kittleson, for a detailed listing of health-related web sites.[4]

Accessing Up-to-Date and State-of-the-Art Health Education Processes

Health educators can use the Internet to access up-to-date information and share it with target populations through their workshop presentations, brochures, flyers, PSAs, and other traditional health education methods. In fact, many sites regularly provide press releases (e.g., American Cancer Society at http://www.cancer.org), action alerts (e.g. American Public Health Association at http://www.apha.org), fact sheets (e.g., Planned Parenthood Federation of America at http://www.igc.apc.org/ppfa/), charts and pictures, and even video PSAs (e.g., CDC's "Respect Yourself,

Protect Yourself" HIV/AIDS prevention at http://www.cdcnac.org/respect.html). For example, action alerts pertaining to pertinent issues (e.g., youth tobacco access) can be accessed from the American Public Health Association's home page. A community coalition could use these alerts to encourage local citizens or legislators to take action for or against a particular issue. In another example, a focus group consisting of representatives of a target population may suggest that a certain type of picture would be effective on the front cover of a brochure. A health educator could conduct a search of the web for a picture that closely matches the suggested image. When located, that picture or image could be easily downloaded to the word processing or desktop publishing document for inclusion in the brochure. Some search engines (e.g., Lycos) provide the ability to search an index of graphics and pictures that exist on the web. Most of these images are available for use with no copyright restrictions. Permission can usually be received for pictures that are copyrighted.

Being connected to the Internet also allows health educators to access state-of-the-art health education processes. Many health educators rely on printed materials such as texts, newspapers, journal articles, and conference proceedings to provide the necessary documentation on new health education models and approaches. Much of this information, however, is dated by the time it appears in print. In the case where a health educator is separated from the mainstream (e.g., health educator in a rural area), opportunities for updates and continued education may be few and far between. In addition to the CDC *Wonder* site, which consists primarily of resource information such as needs assessment data, journal articles, and program abstracts, a number of sites exist that provide health educators with on-line access to state-of-the-art approaches. For instance, the *Community Toolbox* (http://ctb.lsi.ukans.edu) is a site that provides access to "how-to" materials (in addition to links to information, people, funding, and resources) for addressing local health concerns that impact communities (e.g., substance abuse, adolescent pregnancy, youth violence). Health educators can utilize the community development skills outlined at this site to assist in enhancing the communities in which they work. Take, for example, a lone health educator working in a three-county rural health district. In working with a local community's problems, the health educator could access this site via a lap top computer (with a built in modem) connected through a telephone line. By doing so, the health educator would have access to current practices and skills associated with assisting the community in developing effective solutions to deal with its problems. Rather than relying on dated models and knowledge, innovative approaches and problem-solving mechanisms become available. Other resource and technical assistance sites such as *Healthy Cities Online* (http://www.healthycities.org) also exist on the Internet.

Link to Grant Funding Agencies and Foundations

Because external funding has become essential in order for many local health education agencies and organizations to operate, it is imperative to have access to funding sources. Rather than wait for requests for proposals and program announcements to arrive in the mail, health educators need to be proactive in identifying potential funders and funding opportunities. The Internet provides access to numerous agencies and foundations that have funds available. In addition, numerous web sites exist that can assist health educators in writing grants.

Electronic Mail

Within the last few years electronic mail (e-mail) has emerged as a prominent communication vehicle. Prior to the advent of electronic messaging, user communication was dependent on the telephone, postal services and, more recently, fax machines. The advantages associated with e-mail provide a greater latitude than traditional communication vehicles in that e-mail utilizes the Internet structure in order to route messages between users. Each user has an e-mail account that is connected to a domain server. Most of the current Internet browsers contain an application known as an e-mail "client" which provides e-mail access. In addition, a number of sites on the web offer free e-mail (e.g., MailExcite at http://mail.excite.com).

E-mail addresses consist of a user name and the domain to which the user is attached, separated by "@." For instance, the e-mail address for the author of this chapter is *bensley@wmich.edu*. Both the user name (*bensley*) and domain (*wmich.edu*) are specified in the address. Messages sent to this address are routed to the domain associated with *wmich.edu*. Within the domain name is the site (*wmich* which, in this case, stands for *Western Michigan University*) and the structure type of the site (*edu*). Sites are typically educational institutions (edu), government (gov), organizations or associations (org), or commercial companies (com).

Messages can be sent to either single or multiple addresses. This allows for latitude in sharing information with more than one party, scheduling meetings or events, and electronic conference calling. For instance, health educators could use e-mail to schedule committee meetings, share project results with colleagues or funders, submit inquiries to experts in the field, or connect with hard-to-reach individuals. A disadvantage to e-mail is that it is less personable than a telephone call. This is offset by the fact that e-mail has no time restrictions. A message can be sent or responded to at anytime, regardless of time of day or night.

E-mail users also can subscribe to health-related discussion group forums and *listservs*. These groups consist of like-minded e-mail subscribers who connect together for the purpose of sharing information and debating issues. Listservs are an excellent mechanism for problem solving with other professionals. Usually included on a listserv will be experts in the field related to practically every aspect of the issue. Not all listservs operate in this manner though. Some listservs function as an avenue for distributing information to subscribed users. With these listservs, users do not submit messages, but rather are recipients of daily reports. For instance, the listserv AIDSNEWS (listproc@aspensys.com) provides users with a daily AIDS report comprised of statistics, trends, and findings.

Numerous national health-related discussion groups and listservs exist. For example, the *Healthy Cities Online* web site includes a number of discussion forums that are pertinent to aspects of community building. Users can usually subscribe to a listserv by sending a message addressed to the e-mail address of the listserv. The user should leave the subject line blank and within the body of the message include (without quotes) "subscribe listserv-name your-name" where "listserv-name" is the name of the listserv and "your-name" is the user's first and last name (separated by a blank space). For example, the author of this chapter could subscribe to BUSHEA-L, a worksite health promotion listserv, by sending an e-mail message to *listserv@siu.edu* and include in the message text *subscribe bushea-l robert bensley*. A sample of health-related listservs can be found in Table 13-1.

Health educators could use e-mail to establish a local discussion group. This could be accomplished by establishing an alias user name consisting of the addresses for each user in the forum. A message sent to the alias user name would then be received by everyone on the list. Each user would have to create a similar alias. For instance, a health educator working in a rural district may design an information-sharing and problem-solving e-mail group that links together the health education related agencies that exist in each local community. In a similar sense, a health educator could use an e-mail discussion group to link local agencies with agencies from other rural districts, expanding the ability for users to work together, solve problems, and share approaches. At the state level, health educators

Table 13-1. Health-Related Discussion Groups

Listserv Name	Address	Topic
AIDS-L	listserv@siu.edu	HIV/AIDS
BUSHEA-L	listserv@siu.edu	Worksite health promotion
CANCER-L	listserv@wvnvm.bitnet	Cancer
FIT-L	listserv@maelstrom.stjohns.edu	Wellness, exercise, and diet
HEDIR-L	listserv@siu.edu	Health education issues
HEDIRS-L	listserv@siu.edu	University students listserv
HLTHPROM	listserver@relay.doit.wisc.edu	University health promotion

could link local coalitions together via an e-mail discussion group. What is currently being addressed through use of newsletters and summary reports could easily be shared via an e-mail system.

Finally, e-mail becomes an essential tool for distributing documents without the expense or time involved with mailing, faxing, and telephone calling. For instance, e-mail could be used for the timely distribution of an action alert or a letter-writing campaign. Documents and files can easily be attached to an e-mail message and forwarded to any user who has an e-mail address. In order for this approach to work, the targeted audience must have access to e-mail, which is not always the case. At a minimum, users who are connected via e-mail could be separated out and added to an "e-mail action alert list." Even if only a few of the targeted group use e-mail, it still reduces the time and expense of telephone calling and faxing.

Personal Assessment and Behavior Change Applications

Computer programs can be used to increase user awareness of behavioral practices that may be harmful to their health. These applications can consist of a simple series of questions that pertain to either a specific health behavior or a multitude of behaviors. Prior to the infusion of technology, these applications were generally paper and pencil assessments that used predefined scales to categorize respondents based on their responses. Although personal assessment programs are more elementary than more advanced risk-appraisal applications, they still can be useful for increasing awareness about personal health behavior. In addition, they are easy to develop or acquire, and inexpensive. Although most health educators would rather adopt a more complex and useful risk-appraisal program, personal assessment programs can be used when simple awareness is the goal.

Many web sites include a personal assessment program (see Table 13-2 for example sites). Users connected to the Internet can simply access these sites and answer the questions, resulting in an increased awareness of personal health behaviors. A health educator could use an existing web assessment application in order to raise awareness of a target group's behavior. For instance, a health educator who works with nutrition could include a personal assessment web site address (e.g., *CyberDiet's Nutritional Profile* at http://www.cyberdiet.com/index.html) on pamphlets, flyers, and other items that are distributed to the general public at health fairs, community centers, and other resource avenues.

Personal assessment programs can also be interactive. These programs usually operate from a CD-ROM or hard drive on a microcomputer and are designed to guide the user through a learning experience based on their responses to questions about certain behaviors and risk factors. They are unique in the sense that screens are predefined, but are sequenced in

Table 13-2. Web-Based Personal Health Assessments

Assessment Focus	Web Site
Women's health	http://www.womens-health.com
General HRA	http://wellness.uwsp.edu/health_service/services/ lifescan.shtml
General HRA	http://youfirst.com/
Longevity	http://www.northwesternmutual.com/games/ longevity/
Nutrition	http://www.cyberdiet.com/index.html
Stress	http://wellness.uwsp.edu/health_service/services/ stress.shtml
Temperament	http://wellness.uwsp.edu/college_health/
Wellness	http://wellness.uwsp.edu/health_service/services/ livewell/index.shtml

response to the specific answers of each user. In addition to increased awareness of behavioral practices, opportunity for education about specific risks and practices exists. For instance an interactive HIV assessment program (*HIV: Assessing Your Risk*), created by the Office of Health Promotion and Education at Western Michigan University, was designed to assist a university community in learning about HIV/AIDS and personal practices that put them at risk for HIV infection. Users are able to access the interactive program at stations located at the university health center, all of which are set up for complete confidentiality. Preliminary results have been positive and the application currently serves as a national model for HIV/AIDS awareness and education in a university setting. Health educators could develop computer learning stations in STD and other public health clinics, schools, churches, and community centers that use this or other interactive-type programs. An excellent example of such a program is *The Choice is Yours*, an interactive videodisc program that reduces HIV/STD risk by teaching adolescents decision-making skills and socially appropriate responses to potentially risky sexual situations.[5]

Many interactive assessments utilize a referral system in addition to offering personalized health information. For instance, the *Youth Health Provider* assesses the social and behavioral health history of adolescents, covering all issues of preventive care outlined by the *AMA Guidelines for Adolescent Preventive Services*. Based on responses to an interactive health interview, clients are dispensed specific printed take-home materials, provided with problem-specific health advise and local referrals, and administered pertinent health education videos.[6]

Different from personal assessment programs, health risk appraisals (HRAs) are computerized applications that determine the odds of being at risk to morbidity and mortality and assess an individual's future prospects for good health.[7] Almost all HRAs provide individual health projections over the next 10 years by measuring individual risk against national mortality databases and epidemiologically-derived risk estimates. Central to all HRAs is a report that is generated based on user responses. The details of the reports differ with each HRA, but all tend to provide generic recommendations for reducing risk. Many HRAs currently exist, each differing based on the target group for which it is intended. Worksite health promotion specialists use HRAs to assess employee health status on an ongoing basis. Rather than using an HRA only to identify initial risk, it becomes an effective way to assess individual progress in reducing negative health risks.

Computer-tailored messages have been found to be promising in relation to changing client behavior. This procedure involves generating personalized client messages based on responses to a personal assessment program. For instance, the *Interactive Multimedia Health Risk Appraisal* is an interactive touch screen kiosk application that selects tailored video clips for patients based on questions about their medical history and life-style habits.[8] Other programs have found that using computer-tailored letters has been successful with difficult-to-change behaviors such as decreasing fat consumption and smoking.[9,10] Although placement of touch screen kiosks in malls and other high traffic areas could be an effective means of reaching the general public, cost is likely to be prohibitive for most health education agencies. Tailored letters, however, could be developed and mailed, e-mailed, or faxed to all individuals who completed a personal assessment or HRA. For example, with a little help from a computer programmer, a worksite health promotion specialist could tailor a series of letters in response to employee HRAs or personal assessments.

Desktop Publishing and Graphic Art Applications

The introduction of graphic user interface (GUI) technology in the 1980s made it possible to create and manipulate graphical images which previously were done by a graphic artist. Since then, numerous graphical image application programs have been developed to replace much of what the graphic artist used to create free hand. Along with graphical manipulation, GUI technology provided the ability to adjust the leading (space existing between lines) so that typesetting, which had previously been the responsibility of printers and commercial typesetters, could be done on the computer. Because health educators are heavily involved with creating materials that use type and graphical images (e.g., brochures, flyers, newsletters), "desktop publishing" applications have become necessary tools.

Desktop publishing consists of computer programs (e.g., PageMaker, Microsoft Publisher) that allow users to easily manipulate text and images through the process of cutting and pasting. It is different from a traditional word processing program in that the open page is similar to a drawing board where images and text can be placed regardless of tabs and other document layout concerns. In addition, publishing programs allow the user to make proportional adjustments to the leading between lines, providing a professional typeset appearance.

These application programs are used mostly by health educators who are responsible for developing newsletters and other professional printed materials. For example, a health educator could use a desktop publishing application to generate monthly newsletters for a local community coalition. Included could be photographs of local events, graphical images, statistics, summary reports, and other text and image pieces.

In addition to desktop publishing, advanced graphical manipulation applications include graphic art drawing programs (e.g., Quickdraw, FreeHand, Illustrator) and programs that allow the alteration of photographs (e.g., Photoshop). These applications are commonly used by professional graphic artists. A health educator with graphic art skills who has access to these programs can produce extremely high quality materials. As the capability of these programs become more common place, health educators are more likely to seek out the skills needed to be proficient in them.

Presentation Applications

Some software packages are designed to provide an easy-to-use presentation application that can be used to convey information during a public speaking engagement (e.g., PowerPoint). These programs allow the presenter to use text, web pictures, graphics, and even short video movie clips to supplement their presentation. A menu driven system allows the user to develop a number of screens, or "slides," each with the capacity to contain multiple formats (e.g., text, graphics, movie clips), builds, and transitions between slides. During speaking engagements, the presenter uses a mouse to simply "click" the slides forward allowing for better control over the tempo of the presentation.

Health educators can use presentation applications to enhance the quality and effectiveness of speaking engagements, especially those that are more formal in nature. For instance, if presenting to a local governing board (e.g., City Commission, Township Board) to build support for a local community-wide youth violence initiative, statistical graphics, pictures of local youth and violence-related events, sample video clips of PSAs from national campaigns, and impactful builds and transitions are more likely to win support than traditional overheads.

With any computer-generated application, equipment is needed. In particular, the presenter would need a lap top computer to access the presentation, and a projection panel that can fit on an overhead projector. Both of these pieces are relatively small and easy to carry. In fact, all equipment needed (other than the overhead projector) could easily fit into a standard briefcase.

Distance Learning

In the past, it has been difficult for many health educators to find avenues that provided opportunities for continued education. Learning mechanisms primarily consisted of professional journals and conferences. Due to cost, work load and location, many of these opportunities were not feasible for local health educators. As mentioned previously, the advent of the Internet has provided access to a tremendous amount of information. Health educators who are connected to the Internet are able to educate themselves about new and innovative processes. Unfortunately, not all health educators have access to the Internet. Many still fight the "budget battle" in which computer equipment and services are usually not a priority. The development of *distance learning* has provided many local health educators with affordable, accessible opportunities to further their education.

Distance learning is based on the process of transmitting a video presentation from a central site to external sites, via satellite links or phone lines. In order for this type of technology to be used, both the sending and receiving sites need to have the appropriate equipment and be properly wired to make the connection. Most satellite programs are one-way transmissions consisting of national presentations. Two-way audio/visual satellite programs are very rare, because the costs and equipment associated with the uplink (sending) are tremendous—definitely not a budget item that a local nonprofit agency could justify. Many communities, however, have an agency or an organization that has the capability to receive satellite transmission. Universities, hospitals, community colleges, and intermediate school districts are most likely to have this capability. Rather than having to travel to another state in order to attend a workshop, a health educator could travel to a site within their community that is sponsoring a distance-learning event.

National agencies such as CDC frequently sponsor distance learning programming. Many state public health agencies and associations sponsor satellite connection to these national events. Gaining access to state-of-the-art information and processes from national experts is invaluable to a local health educator who would otherwise miss out on the opportunity to receive this information.

Distance learning is most commonly achieved with videoconferencing systems. These are units that send and receive digitally-compressed audio and video signals via telephone lines. What was first envisioned as a way for businesses to conduct face-to-face conferencing from different parts of the world has become a powerful tool for providing workshops and seminars to remote areas. Almost every major university and hospital in the U.S. has the capability to engage in videoconferencing. In addition, this technology also exists in many public schools and businesses. In most cases, videoconferencing is a point-to-point transmission. Some of the more progressive organizations have a video bridge that allows for multi-point videoconferencing. There are services in some major cities that rent out bridge time that enable multiple site connections. In addition, many Internet browsers provide applications that provide access to audio and visual communication from desktop computers, lending great versatility to multi-site conferencing.

Health educators could use videoconferencing to provide interactive workshops to users at remote sites. For example, a community health educator could schedule time with an organization that has videoconferencing capabilities to create an in-service program geared toward remote health educators. Those invited could attend one of a number of remote sites (the number of sites would be dependent on the capability of the bridge) with access to videoconferencing technology. This becomes a cost efficient approach to sharing information, especially if distance is a consideration.

Data Analysis Applications

As all statistical analysts can attest to, a computer is a necessary component of any research project. The complexity of statistical analysis is such that most advanced data analysis methods are nearly impossible to complete without a computer program. Thankfully, numerous data analysis programs exist (e.g., SPSS, SAS) with some being reasonable in cost. In general, all programs are similar and contain basic and advanced statistical methods. One particular program, *Epi Info*, is a public domain program (available from CDC at http://www.cdc.gov/epo/epi/epiinfo.htm) that has been popular with public health educators. *Epi Info* is a series of computer programs that aide in manipulating epidemiological data in questionnaire format and organizing study designs and results in text as part of a written report. Included are features for creating databases, analyzing data, and reporting results. This program could be used by a health educator responsible for collecting and reporting epidemiological data, such as that found in a community health assessment and improvement project.

Computer programs are also available to assist practitioners in the assessment, planning, implementation, and evaluation phases of health education programming. For example, *EMPOWER* is a computerized program designed to assist practitioners in their efforts to plan, implement, and assess the outcome of community-based health promotion programs, especially mammography screenings. Based on the PRECEDE/PROCEED planning process, *EMPOWER* provides access to models and interventions for breast cancer prevention and control. Encompassed in the program is an extensive decision-support system, which produces recommended action steps. A local health educator could use this program to assist in developing and evaluating a community-wide program aimed at impacting early breast cancer detection efforts.

Program Management Applications

A number of computer applications can be used to assist health educators in the day-to-day management of their programs. These applications are typically referred to as "office" programs and consist of word processing, spreadsheet, calendaring, and project management programs. Word processing programs (e.g., Word and Word Perfect) provides health educators with the capability to compose letters, documents, reports, flyers, faxes, and even brochures and newsletters. Spreadsheet programs (e.g., Excel and Lotus 1-2-3) provide the capability to organize and manipulate data, whether in the form of a (e.g.) budget, chart, or schedule of events. Calendaring programs allow users to easily manage time schedules. Project management programs (e.g., Microsoft Project) provide users with the ability to plan, manage, and track the progress of projects. As these applications are generally commonplace among most computer systems and because their application is not difficult to understand (e.g., using word processing to create a thank you letter, using a spreadsheet to develop a budget), they will not be covered further in this chapter. Numerous books, self-help guides, community classes, and tutorials are available to assist the reader in further expanding knowledge with these applications.

BARRIERS TO USING TECHNOLOGY

It is true with most health educators that what appears to makes sense, such as the infusion of technology into health education processes, is easier said than done. There are a number of barriers that impede the progression from the use of traditional health education delivery mechanisms to more advanced technological approaches. Just because technology is available does not mean that it will, or should, always be used. Hopefully, however, the reasons for incorporating technology can be justified. It may take time to overcome the barriers listed in this section. No need to worry. It took 6,000-plus years to reach the point at which we currently are.

Factors that hinder the effective implementation of technology into health education processes include the following:

- *Cost and lack of equipment.* There is no question that technology is expensive. For some approaches, the cost can be enormous. Being a nonprofit driven service industry, most health education agencies are under financial constraints and do not have the funds necessary to purchase technologically-advanced equipment and materials. There tends to be a belief that funds should be spent directly on the services provided to the target population, rather than the mechanisms necessary for ensuring that these services are impactful. To complicate matters, many areas (especially those that are rural) do not yet have physical access to even the simplest technology such as cellular phones or local Internet connection.

- *Target population lack of access to technology.* Although the Internet has become common place in society, many still do not have access to it. As the Internet is currently the technology avenue for the future, target populations need to somehow gain access to it.

- *Agency lack of support for technology.* Even those agencies that have suitable equipment do not always have the structure in place to educate staff on how to use available technology or to continually upgrade existing equipment and programs. Health educators are not computer scientists. They generally need assistance in determining what equipment is needed and how to use it.

- *Target population lack of knowledge.* Not only do target populations lack access to technology, many lack the knowledge necessary in order to make effective use of it. It may seem appropriate to list web sites on a brochure with the anticipation that readers will be motivated to review the site. Many have never even touched a computer and are, therefore, less likely to comply with the recommendation.

- *Target population unwillingness to change.* People in general do not enjoy change. Most would rather stay at the current level in which they function because to move forward would require change. This is especially true in the ever-changing, hard-to-grasp world of technology.

- *Lack of human presence.* One of the greatest complaints of using technology is that it lacks a human element. This sometimes is the trade-off for having access to technology. Most individuals would rather have a person to talk with about a problem than a machine. Because of the nature of the issues with which health educators work, the lack of human interaction may not always be the best course of action. Therefore, it is important that health educators use technology to *supplement*, rather than supplant, their efforts.

- *Quality and accuracy of web sites.* The Internet has grown exponentially. With this growth, it is near impossible to continually evaluate all new web sites for accuracy and quality. Just because the information exists on the web does not mean that it is credible or appropriate. This is most evident with the current debate over the multitude of pornographic sites that exist on the web. At some point, a system may be established for reviewing the accuracy and appropriateness of web sites. Until then, health educators need to be able to determine the credibility of sites. Many resources for evaluating web sites currently exist. In particular, the reader is referred to "Evaluating Health-Related Web Sites" by Lisa Pealer and Steve Dorman, "Evaluation of Web Resources" at http://cyclops.idbsu.edu/quality.htm, *Web Sites for Health Professionals* by Mark Kittleson, and the Purdue University Libraries web site evaluation page located at http://thorplus.lib.purdue.edu/~techman/eval.html.[4,11]

- *Current methods are not designed with technology and the future in mind.* For various reasons, many health educators continue to focus on traditional programming and refuse to explore the potential associated with incorporating advanced technology. Survey research continues to rely heavily on the U.S. postal system, presenters carry chalk and transparency markers with them, and health educators gather resources from agency libraries consisting of dated journals and texts. Budgets are done on paper sheets and brochures are a mixture of word processing and literal cutting and pasting of images. Not only do these methods fail to take advantage of the available technology, they make it nearly impossible to use as a base for future adaptations. For example, a brochure that has been physically cut and pasted leaves little room for additional changes to meet future needs. Wasted effort is used in recreating the product. In contrast, a brochure that was developed using desktop publishing can be modified and changed with relatively little effort.

STRATEGIES FOR OVERCOMING BARRIERS

While it is not always easy to overcome the aforementioned barriers, health educators should make every effort to incorporate technology into their practices. It can be done. The following suggestions can aid in reducing the impact of those barriers:

- *Securing grant funding and donations.* Actively pursuing and securing grant funding can provide the finances needed to interject technology into health education practices. As presented in Chapter 12 ("Grant Writing"), some foundations and local organizations provide capital expenditure grants that support the acquisition of equipment. Local organizations and businesses may also have equipment that could be donated to nonprofit agencies. Although the technology may be a year or two old, it is something with which to get started. Because the cost of computer software and upgrades is fairly inexpensive, donated equipment may be able to brought up to speed at a fraction of the cost of purchasing new products. Most state and federal grants do not support the purchase of equipment unless the proposed project cannot operate without it. Partnering with schools or other local agencies may increase the likelihood that funders would be willing to invest in technology.

- *Tapping into resources available at institutions of higher learning.* Many communities have access to a local or state college or university. Because of the academic and research nature of colleges and universities, they can be excellent resources for assisting local agencies and communities in designing plans for technology infusion. Within these institutions are highly trained researchers and professionals who can act as consultants, assist in planning workshops and in-services, provide access to advanced technology, serve as distance learning bridge sites, and provide the research and evaluation expertise needed for securing grant funding. As many college and university personnel are involved with professional health education associations, they can have a great impact on establishing protocols to ensure the future use of technology is both ethical and credible.

- *Providing education and in-servicing.* The profession needs to continue to sponsor conferences and workshops designed to aid other health educators in keeping up to speed with the application of technology. Many professional conferences already provide sessions on infusion of technology in practice. In addition, many professional journals have devoted entire issues to technology applications in health education. As health educators become more adept at using available technology, they must ensure that it is being infused into practice. The use of technology to enhance personal health (e.g., using web site personal assessment applications to identify health practices) can be spread through speaking engagements at PTA meetings, churches, schools, community centers, and worksites. Target populations need to be made aware of where and how they can access technology (e.g., most community libraries have a dedicated computer station that is connected to the Internet).

- *Infusing technology into community resource centers.* In addition to library access to the Internet, other community centers (e.g., Boys and Girls Club, neighborhood associations, YMCAs, schools, churches) should be encouraged to provide access to the Internet for their patrons. Most will likely say that funds are not available for that type of service. An innovative grant proposal justifying that the use of community-wide technology improves key community health indicators may justify the costs.

CONCLUSION

The benefits associated with utilizing technology are many. Most importantly, technology will provide broader access to populations at risk, increase professionalism among health educators, result in the infusion of innovative approaches to solving negative health behaviors, and provide timely access to state-of-the-art information and processes. In order to experience these benefits, however, it takes time, patience, energy, and determination.

Health educators are currently in the midst of change. A shift is occurring where we can no longer depend on traditional tools and methods for enacting change in community norms and behaviors. Health educators must seek out, embrace, and understand how to make the best use of technological advances that occur daily. The future is near. With it will come greater use of concepts such as virtual reality and home-communication stations (e.g., a combined computer, television, and telephone device). Either we can run from it, or embrace it for the good of all. Regardless, it is here to stay.

References

1. Daniel, E. L., & Balog, J. E. (1997). Utilization of the world wide web in health education. *Journal of Health Education, 28*, 260-267.

2. Pealer, L. N. (1996). Computer communications technology and the future of health education. *The Health Education Monograph Series, 14*(2), 26-29.

3. Kotecki, J. E., & Siegel, D. (1997). Finding health information via the world wide web: An essential resource for the community health practitioner. *Journal of Health Education, 28,* 117-120.

4. Kittleson, M. J. (1997). *Web sites for health professionals.* Sudbury, MA: Jones and Bartlett Publishers.

5. Noell, J., Ary, D., & Duncan, T. (1997). Development and evaluation of a sexual decision-making and social skills program: "The Choice is YoursæPreventing HIV/STDs." *Health Education & Behavior, 24,* 87-101.

6. Paperny, D. M. N. (1997). Computerized health assessment and education for adolescent HIV and STD prevention in health care settings and schools. *Health Education & Behavior, 24,* 54-70.

7. Dunton, S. (1991). An introduction to health risk appraisals at the workplace. In J. P. Mayer & J. K. David (Eds.), *Worksite health promotion: Needs, approaches, and effectiveness* (Chapter 2). Lansing, MI: Michigan Department of Public Health.

8. Irvine, B., Beauchamp, N., & Wells, J. (1997). Interactive health risk appraisal for behavior change (Practice notes: Strategies in health education). *Health Education & Behavior, 24,* 8-9.

9. Brug, J., Steenhuis, I., van Assema, P., & de Vries, H. (1996). The impact of a computer-tailored nutrition intervention, *Preventive Medicine, 25,* 236-242.

10. Strecher, V. J., Kreuter, M., Boer, D., Kobrin, S., Hospers, H. J., & Skinner, C. S. (1994). The effects of computer-tailored smoking cessation messages in family practice settings. *Journal of Family Practice, 39,* 262-270.

11. Pealer, L. N., & Dorman, S. M. (1997). Evaluating health-related web sites. *Journal of School Health, 67,* 232-235.

Chapter 14

PROMOTING MULTICULTURAL DIVERSITY

Jodi Brookins-Fisher, Ph.D., C.H.E.S.

Author's Comment: *I really feel that relating to people on a human level is the most important thing we can do to make a difference in people's lives. How are we to develop and implement effective programs if we do not know the people with which we are working? It seems so basic, yet it is a point that has been overlooked for years. The focus on diversity is long overdue. We need to realize and validate the important differences in people. They should not have to be like "me" in order to receive services in this country. Unfortunately, just the opposite is often true.*

    *This chapter addresses diversity from a practical perspective. But beyond that, we need to realize diversity in health education because it is the **human** thing to do. We should all be able to enjoy our health because we are citizens of a great country—not because of our skin color, sexual orientation, or age. Health educators can make the world a better place and we can begin by acknowledging all of the people that make up its uniqueness.*

INTRODUCTION

In the last few years, an increased emphasis on the inclusion of diverse cultures in America has played a major role in health education efforts. These community-based efforts have been initiated in response to increases in disease among particular populations (e.g., stroke among African-Americans). With changes in programming, an understanding of concepts such as "cultural awareness," "cultural sensitivity," "cultural competence," and "multiculturalism" have become necessary for a health educator to be effective. It is easy to give terminology lip service, but what do these terms really mean? What must the health education profession do to encompass the issues of diversity in the many settings in which it is a part? How would an individual health educator become better prepared to work with diversity? This chapter addresses the need for a multicultural focus in health education, presents ideas on how to develop a multicultural setting and how to overcome barriers, and lists diversity awareness resources available to health educators.

The Need for Multicultural Awareness in Health Education

From an ethnic and racial standpoint, the United States population is changing from one that is largely Caucasian, to one that is more diverse. It has been projected that by the year 2030, the ethnic group with the largest percentage of increase in population will be Hispanic-Americans, equating to a 187% increase. It is also projected that during the same time, Asian-American, Pacific Islander-American, and Native-American populations will each experience a 79% increase, and African-Americans will experience a 68% population growth. In contrast, only a 25% increase will occur among Caucasians. The projected population increases will change the overall percentages that each of these groups constitute in the U.S., so that "minority" ethnic groups, collectively, will surpass the Caucasian population in numbers, accounting for 51% of the population. This shift will result in the U.S. being more similar to global statistics, in which people of color comprise the "majority."

Other demographic indicators also demonstrate growing multiculturalism in America. By the year 2000, one-fifth of the U.S. population will be over the age of 65, with individuals over 85 years being the fastest growing population in America. Additionally, studies suggest that gay and lesbian persons currently represent 10-15% of the U.S. population.

Therefore, it is essential that health education, in both the present and the future, continues to be aware of and respond to demographic changes. Growing "minority" populations will need services attuned to cultural considerations. Regardless of the specific population to be targeted, the development of health education services will need to include the population's culture in community health assessment and improvement, program planning, implementation, and evaluation.

One consistent factor is that U.S. populations will continue to experience problems with certain health issues. For example, poverty, lack of proper immunizations, heart disease, cancer, stroke, chronic obstructive pulmonary disease, pneumonia, and diabetes will continue to plague ethnic groups, while older adults will continue to experience chronic diseases, such as arthritis, hypertension, osteoporosis, and dementing illnesses.[1] As the country's demographics change, it is imperative that health educators provide programming that addresses the largest health concerns of their diverse populations.

The Language of Diversity

Terminology pertaining to multiculturalism abounds:

- *Diversity* refers to divergence or deviation among people, rooted in age, culture, health status and condition, ethnicity, experience, gender, sexual orientation, and various combinations of these traits.

- *Cultural awareness* is the consciousness of cultural similarities and differences.[2]

- *Cultural sensitivity* has been described as "the knowledge that cultural differences exist."[2]

- *Cultural competence* is a "characteristic of those individuals who hold academic and interpersonal skills which allow an increased understanding and appreciation of another group's differences and similarities."[1] Culturally competent individuals have made an effort to learn about other cultures and have incorporated the information to the point where assumptions about others are not made. Other definitions of cultural competence have included institutions, systems, and practitioners, with the ultimate result being the ability to respond to the unique needs of populations that differ from the majority, mainstream culture.[3]

- *Multiculturalism* has been defined as a recognition of racial and cultural diversity, respect for the beliefs and culture of others, and a recognition that all members of a society have contributions to make for its betterment.[4] It includes the concept of equality among peoples regardless of such concepts as race, ethnicity, gender, sexual orientation, age, or ability. In addition, multiculturalism can be both a vocabulary term and a phenomenon at the individual or institutional level; inclusive of cultures outside of the majority.[5]

Multiculturalism has also been applied to education. The term *multicultural education* has been developed to refer to "the process of gaining an enhanced understanding, acceptance, and knowledge of the methods of constructive interactions among people of differing cultural backgrounds."[5] Within the health education profession, *multicultural health education* has been defined as learning opportunities designed with sensitivity to culture, values, beliefs, and practices that are carried out in relevant languages. These educational activities are developed and implemented with the active participation of people reflective of the target population, and take into account their cultural diversity.[6]

While society has gotten itself wrapped up in the muddied waters of "political correctness," the present and future of the health education profession will require an understanding of multicultural issues beyond "correctness." For health education practitioners, the importance lies deeper than that of learning the language, it lies in the importance of equalizing the playing field for all players. The profession could pride itself in knowing the terminology, but if health education does not contribute to change in societal structure for the betterment of all peoples, it will be missing a critical component of the profession for the 21st century.

DEVELOPING A MULTICULTURAL SETTING

Personal Awareness

Before developing and implementing programs for diverse populations, health educators must first understand their own belief systems regarding issues of diversity (e.g., race, ethnicity, religion, gender, sexual orientation, age, ability). The first step in this process involves becoming familiar with personal biases. Health educators need to be in touch with their personal biases, so that they do not disrupt services and education provided in cross-cultural or transcultural (i.e., experiences with others different from oneself) settings. People have different experiencesæthey naturally bring judgments to any interaction with people different than themselves. Social experiences with other groups, political interactions, and communication and problem-solving patterns can all impact interactions with others, and lead to stereotypes and misunderstanding.[4] By understanding personal biases, health educators will be better able and more confident in communicating with target populations.

Health educators also must determine if their personal biases can be separated from professional interactions. Even though all humans naturally have biases, health educators must make every effort not to bring their biases into professional settings, as this will affect their abilities to work with diverse populations. This is a difficult task, and one that should be carefully analyzed prior to programming at any level.

Along with careful evaluation of personal biases, the importance of reading, participating, watching, and listening cannot be underestimated in becoming a culturally competent professional. Health educators can learn the most about other cultures when they allow themselves to be immersed in the cultures of other populations. Ideas for learning about other cultures include (1) attending cultural events, such as Pride Day, Cinco de Mayo, or ethnic celebrations; (2) participating in workshops or lectures about topics on different cultures; (3) being involved in other neighborhood activities in the community; and (4) reading materials from people of different cultural backgrounds. The importance of establishing relationships with people from different cultures is, perhaps, the most beneficial way to learn about their cultures. These relationships will allow free discussion and provide opportunities to listen and learn from other points of view.

Transferring Personal Knowledge Into Professional Settings

Once awareness of personal biases has increased, knowledge learned about other cultures should be transferred into both professional practice and the workplace. At a broader professional level, the following strategies can enhance a health educator's ability to understand diversity, and help ensure that it is incorporated into professional practice and workplace interactions:[4]

- Determine whether current expertise addresses both local and worldwide diversity and responsibility for humankind and international interactions.

- Determine whether programs enhance people's skills and knowledge about the diverse world around them, to better understand themselves and the values of other cultures.

- Determine whether materials, curricula, services, and resources benefit all target populations. Materials should reflect gender, racial, and other cultural equities (e.g., gender-neutral language).

- Determine whether an action plan has been developed relating to special information for underserved populations, such as migrant farm workers, immigrants, and homeless persons.

- Determine whether plans incorporating *Healthy People 2000* into programming have also included the needs of diverse populations.

- Develop an evaluation mechanism that measures the extent to which the health education workplace is meeting multicultural responsibilities.

By evaluating the above components, the health educator will begin to determine the cultural competence of the professional setting. Once these items have been analyzed, an organization will know its strengths, weaknesses, and areas for improvement in both the workplace and programming.

Creating an Inclusive Environment

Creating an educational environment inclusive of the diversity among participants can be one of the greatest challenges in health education programming. Several areas of concern will need to be addressed, including (1) the use of language, (2) understanding of the target population culture, (3) discussion guidelines, (4) facilitation skills, (5) use of materials, and (6) teaching techniques and learning styles.

Language

Health educators should remember the importance of inclusive language when presenting information. Language is one of the most important methods for communicating, yet can be the hardest to change for inclusiveness. Both oral and written communication must be clearly understood by diverse populations. Strategies for ensuring inclusiveness include oral and written communication that is gender neutral (e.g., use of the word "partner," "spokesperson"), in the appropriate language, and at the appropriate literacy level. Reading level analysis programs and learner verification procedures should be used with written materials. If materials will be developed in different languages, members of the target community should be involved. Pictures and words conveying health messages should be used where appropriate. If language issues are not considered, health educators risk not connecting with the target population at the most basic level.

Understanding the Target Population Culture

Another area of challenge is becoming aware of the culture of the target population. It is very difficult to understand a population's culture if it has not been experienced by someone living outside the cultural parameters. Culture in itself is diverse, and generalizations will not necessarily hold true for any particular target population. Health educators should participate in cultural events, find the target population's cultural uniqueness by immersing themselves in the community, and establish relationships with people in the target population prior to program implementation. Even when the health educator is properly prepared, cross-cultural interactions may include previous experiences of the participants that may impede the educational process. Although this may be frustrating, the health educator should remain motivated and interested in participants' points of view. If needed, community resources and organizations that are cultural-specific are great resources for troubleshooting problematic areas.

Discussion Guidelines

Group discussion guidelines (e.g., focus groups, classes) should also be determined and stated at the beginning of any program or event, and should be maintained by the facilitator and group members. Discussions among groups should be sensitive to diversity. Guidelines for inclusiveness may include any, or all of the following: (1) Respecting confidentiality of all participants' comments and actions, (2) being sensitive to different personal experiences of group members, (3) being sensitive to different levels of expertise among the group, (4) avoiding assumptions about the cultural/ethnic backgrounds of other group members, (5) allowing privacy (i.e., the right to pass in any discussion or activity), and (6) other guidelines that the group deems important in order to facilitate tolerance and respect for each person's point of view.

Facilitation Skills

Health educators should be facilitators of acceptance and respect in any setting. Good facilitation skills require negotiation, the ability to deal with controversy, being approachable and open, and being objective and impartial. If proper facilitation occurs, a health educator can be a role model for inclusiveness.

Use of Materials

When determining which materials to include in programming, an effort should be made to select pieces from many perspectives. For instance, articles by women and people of color can culturalize a curriculum. By remembering there is diversity among participants, health educators will utilize materials from more than one viewpoint.

Teaching Techniques and Learning Styles

It is always easiest to teach how one prefers to be taught, but this may not reach all participants. Educating should include various methods (e.g., lecture, small groups, role plays, computer exercises) in order to be inclusive of the various learning styles among participants. Because learners may be visual-, tactile-, or audio-oriented, a variety of teaching methods should be incorporated to accommodate different preferences. Values clarification exercises are also valuable in heightening cultural sensitivity, as these help further participant awareness of personal values, while allowing others to state their values. As stated by Noreen Clark, Dean of the School of Public Health at the University of Michigan:[7]

> As a society we have to get agreements on what is important, what we value. .... It's not a matter of your values being better than mine... it's a matter of creating a society where both our values can coexist.

TIPS FOR INCORPORATING MULTICULTURALISM INTO PROFESSIONAL PRACTICE

Take Small Steps Toward Change

As with any other type of behavior change, becoming a culturally competent health educator will take time. Old habits are hard to break, so effort must be made to institute change. It is important to remain oneself throughout the process, as humanness in the effort of trying to be culturally sensitive is an admirable quality. People will be aware of a fake persona anyway, so truth is the best policy. Additionally, as small steps are taken toward inclusiveness, a trust in others must be established. Each client or participant is a unique individual, so care should be taken to not judge based on past experiences. With each successful venture at attaining cultural sensitivity, the health educator will become more culturally competent (see Table 14-1 for traits of a culturally competent health educator).[4]

Practice Facilitation Skills

Although the information presented in Table 14-1 will help equip the health educator with facilitation skills, other tips are also important.[4] Cultural differences can be brought into the discussion through a planned activity regarding a health topic. For example, special remedies for dealing with common illnesses might be discussed, or ethnic foods might be evaluated for nutritional content. By providing these types of opportunities, health educators are encouraging expression of, and acceptance for, cultural differences. Also, the health educator must look at the perspectives of others as a facilitator. Participants may disagree on a concept being presented. As the facilitator, the health educator should be careful to not support or oppose one view. By being open in discussions, the health educator establishes a climate of caring and acceptance. Inclusive language and use of variety in examples will also help facilitation.

Table 14-1. Traits of a Culturally Competent Health Educator

Skills
- Ability to openly discuss racial, ethnic, and other cultural differences and issues.
- Ability to discuss the meaning ethnicity has for the individual person.
- Ability to recognize and combat racism, sexism, ableism, ageism, homophobia, heterosexism, stereotypes, and myths regarding individuals and institutions.
- Ability to evaluate new techniques, research, and knowledge as to their validity and applicability in working with diverse populations.

Personal Attributes
- Concern, empathy, respect, and nonpatronizing support and acceptance.
- A recognition of differences between people.
- Desire and willingness to work with different groups of people.
- Examination and classification of personal values, stereotypes, and biases regarding other groups, and social classes.
- Personal commitment to change "ism's" (e.g., racism, heterosexism).

Knowledge
- Knowledge of other cultures with respect to history, traditions, values, family systems, artistic expression, and the like.
- Knowledge of the help-seeking behavior of other groups of people, including diffusion of information.
- Knowledge of the role of language, special patterns, and communication styles in ethnically distinct communities or settings.
- Recognition of the ways that professional values may conflict with or accommodate the needs of diverse populations.

Know Limits

Being human, health educators may find at times that personal values intrude in professional settings. If this continues, it is always most professional to refer clients to another competent professional that is better able to deal with the issue. This is not to say the health educator should give up, as continued effort may help to work through conflicting personal values and professional obligations.

STRATEGIES FOR OVERCOMING BARRIERS

Personal Barriers

At the personal level, perhaps the biggest barrier to attaining cultural competence is a lack of awareness. Getting beyond one's paradigm and life focus is difficult, and can only occur when awareness is first heightened. Awareness at a global level encourages sharing of wealth, prosperity, and economic development among all U.S. citizens. It is a difficult process, as expressed in the following sentiments:[8]

> *Simply put, at a time when the economy is weak and many politicians are employing old strategies of blaming minorities for getting more than their fair share, it is not difficult to understand the resistance that many people express toward texts and programs, that, in their minds, merely 'rewrite' history. For these people, all this talk of multiculturalism is little more than an attempt to create a narrative that makes them less than heroic by virtue of acknowledging the significance of others, others who have been oppressed and who have been hitherto viewed not as important but rather as problematic. Because of this, educators cannot underestimate the importance of the reevaluation of the status of individuals and groups of people: Many will be compelled to see their own significance challenged, if not threatened with erasure, as others gain a new place in both texts and the nation.*

Other personal barriers involve value and belief systems, and discomfort, which have been previously discussed. By first becoming aware, other potential barriers will be challenged.

In dealing with personal barriers, the health educator should adhere to professional codes of ethics. The Society for Public Health Education (SOPHE) Code of Ethics includes the importance of inclusion of underserved populations in health education programming (Article II, Section 2).[9] The American Association of Health Education also has a similar code of ethics for health education practice.[10] By following a code of ethics, health educators will ensure they are abiding by professional expectations, versus personal beliefs, when conflict occurs.

Reviewing literature in related disciplines may also help a health educator increase cultural awareness. Although a paucity of information on multiculturalism in health education exists, the reader is referred to Marin and colleagues[1] and Buckner[4] for more information on the importance of cultural diversity in health education programming.

Lastly, to combat any personal resistance, the health educator can refer to several organizations and resources that can help professionals become more cultural aware and competent (See Tables 14-2 and 14-3).

Professional Barriers

In the health education field, the largest barriers to multiculturalism confronting professionals are a lack of research, available health education programming specifically targeting diverse populations, and pre-professional training. Much of the research done in health-related fields has predominantly used Caucasian males as the point of reference. Additionally, research has shown that traditional health education approaches are not as effective with underserved groups of people as with the rest of the population.[1] Last, few professionally trained health educators have received education regarding multicultural issues, as few programs nationally have incorporated a multicultural emphasis in their course content. These barriers may affect a health educator's ability to effectively work with the many diverse target populations for which programs are designed.

Even in a profession in which most individuals consider themselves open-minded, the road to cultural competence has been slow. It is impor-

Table 14-2. Organizations Promoting Multicultural Health Education

American Association for Health Education
1900 Association Drive, Reston, VA 20191-1599, 1-800-321-0789
(Specifically, two publications exist: (1) *Cultural Awareness and Sensitivity: Guidelines for Health Educators,* and (2) *Cultural Awareness and Sensitivity: Resources for Health Educators.*)

American Public Health Association
1015 15th Street NW, Washington, DC 20005, 1-202-789-5600
(APHA has specific caucuses to address diversity issues)

American School Health Association
7263 State Route 43/PO Box 708, Kent, OH 44240, 1-330-678-1601

Society for Public Health Education
1015 15th Street NW, Suite 410, Washington, DC, 20005, 1-202-408-9804

Table 14-3. Resources Promoting Multicultural Health Education

- Banks, J. A. (1997). *Teaching strategies for ethnic studies, sixth edition.* Needham Heights, MA: Allyn & Bacon.

- Banks, J. A., & McGee-Banks, C. A. (1997). *Multicultural education: Issues, and perspectives* (3rd ed.). Needham Heights, MA: Allyn & Bacon.

- Brainard, J. M. (1996). *Cultural diversity in the health classroom.* New York: Glencoe.

- Doyle, E. I. (1995). *In the rough: A teaching strategies directory for cultural diversity in health education.* Denton, TX: Texas Woman's University.

- Gordon, A., & Williams-Brown, K. (1996). *Guiding young children in a diverse society.* Needham Heights, MA: Allyn & Bacon.

- Hopkins-Kavanagh, K., & Kennedy, P. H. (1992). *Promoting cultural diversity: Strategies for health care professionals.* Newbury Park, CA: Sage Publications.

- Matiella, A. C. (1991). *Positively different: Creating a bias-free environment for young children.* Santa Cruz, CA: ETR Associates.

- Randall-David, E. (1989). *Strategies for working with culturally diverse communities and clients.* U.S. Department of Health and Human Services, Bureau of Maternal and Child Health and Resources Development, The Association for the Care of Children's Health.

- Spector, R. E. (1996). *Cultural diversity in health & illness* (4th ed.). Stamford, CT: Appleton & Lange.

tant to be proactive as a profession versus reactive. At the institutional level, health care systems can avoid barriers by (1) being aware and accepting of cultural differences and similarities; (2) having the ability for cultural self-assessment (i.e., how culturally competent the organization is); (3) having the required awareness, understanding, and knowledge of target populations; (4) developing skills that facilitate diversity; and (5) being sensitive to dynamics inherent with cultural interaction.[1]

To improve the status of research regarding multicultural issues in health education, more researchers need to see cultural diversity as important. For instance, a recent study found that only 78 titles of 774 articles that appeared in prominent health education journals eluded to a multicultural emphasis.[11] More research projects will need to be target-population specific, and must be run by adequately trained health educators. It has been recommended that in order to avoid barriers to multiculturalism, professional research should adhere to a number of guidelines including the following:[1]

- Demographic information must be collected on all target populations.

- Better means of reaching underserved populations through interventions must be developed and implemented.

- Peer education must be utilized.

- Studies need to include not only health problems, but social and contextual indicators of their incidence and prevalence.

- Long-term effects of interventions need to be evaluated, as well as programmatic process and impact.

Approaches that are more useful in helping underserved populations than traditional health education programs include peer education, lay health workers (e.g., family members, significant others in the communities), interaction with health care providers, self-help groups, and school-based interventions. When implementing any of these approaches, it is important that cultural issues are addressed by including the values, expectancies, norms, beliefs, and behavioral preferences of the target group.[1]

Along with a multicultural focus, a mind set of advocacy must be instilled in professionally prepared health educators, as they will be in positions to work with people (e.g., administrators, legislators) that have a profound impact on other groups' causes. Colleges and universities training future health educators should incorporate skill building and training on community organization and empowerment, advocacy, volunteerism, and diversity, to prepare students for the realities of changing demographics. Developing culturally sensitive programs will increase the level of culturally competent health educators.

Community Resistance

Community resistance may also be a barrier, especially when dealing with multicultural issues that ignite debates among those with different value systems. For example, inclusion of a gay and lesbian youth support program in a school district may initiate controversy, due to differing belief systems among educators, administrators, parents, and students. Religious values and a lack of information about an issue may also contribute to the resistance.

It is important to be able to handle community opposition to multicultural programming should it occur. Opposition to multicultural programming may even include the target population itself. For example, a Native-American population that has had negative past experiences with health education programs may not be supportive of additional programming. Finding out why they feel as they do, and making sure the program is developed incorporating their perspective, will increase the likelihood of program success.

Overcoming community opposition can be accomplished by developing relationships with key individuals and organizations associated with the target population. These key individuals and groups will provide insight into community norms, values, and belief systems. By believing in what the agency is trying to accomplish, they will help the health educator create a successful plan.

Whenever possible and appropriate, coalitions or partnerships around a particular health issue should be developed. By beginning with a common point of interest (i.e., the health issue), individuals will focus on the issue at hand rather than individual biases about the target population. For example, if a coalition is organized to promote sexual abstinence, including abstinence among gay youth, the group should focus on the issue at hand, instead of personal views about homosexuality. When developing coalitions, the target population and representative organizations must be present to ensure cultural values and beliefs have been included.

It is always better for a program to work with the opposition versus excluding them. By finding a common concept for agreement (e.g., reducing risks to a specific disease), barriers such as conflicting values and personal stereotypes will begin to break down. An attempt at working together shows empathy and concern on the health educator's part. Once the opposition is heard, they may be satisfied and no longer be a program threat. Some groups, however, will refuse to agree with other positions and will not be willing to compromise. When this occurs, partnerships will not likely work for either party involved.

EXPECTED OUTCOMES

By following the above suggestions, health educators can expect to enhance cultural competency. This, in turn, will lead to more culturally-competent institutions, organizations, programs, and research. By including the target population throughout program development, materials and resources will be inclusive of their point of view and more likely utilized in the future.

Another outcome will be mutual trust and respect between groups that traditionally have had turbulent relationships. Many minority groups distrust the mor dominant, or majority, populations (i.e., those populations with power in the social structure) and their services. By ensuring cultural diversity in programming, relationships can be rebuilt with mutual understanding.

Perhaps the greatest outcome will be a health education program that is embraced by the community, to the extent that it is institutionalized by the target population. Because the target population was empowered and included in the process, they will be more likely to take ownership and incorporate the information following the completion of the initial program.

At the personal, professional, and community levels, greater awareness of diversity issues will be obtained, paving the way for new directions in programming for diverse populations. The goal of multicultural diversity can best be summarized by the following:[7]

> We (health educators) have to begin with developing an awareness and knowledge of culture which implies a non-judgmental acceptance of the worth of all ethnic groups—a willingness to see people as much as human beings as members of a particular group... the final stage is to be able to perform a specific task while taking culture into account such that the outcome is better than it would have been had the role of the client's culture not been considered.

CONCLUSION

Society demographics are changing, which directly impacts the practice of health educators. New strategies need to be inclusive of cultural diversity and should be implemented by culturally competent health educators. The health education profession must continue to examine its professional preparation programs, research, literature, programming and curricula, methods, and evaluation strategies to ensure the inclusion of cultural diversity. As stated by Buckner:[4]

> The reality . . . of the 21st century leaves us no alternatives but to be prepared, to be innovative, to be progressive, to be flexible and to dare to meet the challenge of building bridges for our [clients] into the next century.

References

1.   Marin, G., Burhannsstipanov, L., Connell, C. M., Gielen, A. C., Helitzer-Allen, D., Lorig, K., Morisky, D. E., Tenney, M., & Thomas, S. (1995). A research agenda for health education among underserved populations. *Health Education Quarterly, 22,* 346-363.

2.   Redican, K., Stewart, S. H., Johnson, L. E., & Frazee, A. M. (1994). Professional preparation in cultural awareness and sensitivity in health education: A national survey. *Journal of Health Education, 25,* 215-217.

3.   National Alliance of Black School Educators. (1984). *Saving the African-American child.* Author.

4.   Buckner Jr., W. P. (1994). Promoting multicultural sensitivity among educators. *The Comprehensive School Health Challenge* (Vol. 2), (pp. 661-686). Santa Cruz, CA: ETR Associates.

5. Staddon, D. T. (1992). *Multicultural resource manual*. Mt. Pleasant, MI: Central Michigan University Printing Services.

6. MacDonald, J. L., Thompson, P. R., & DeSouza, H. (1988). Multicultural health education: An emerging reality in Canada. *Hygiene, 7*, 12-16.

7. Clark, N. M. (1994). Health educators and the future: Lead, follow, or get out of the way. *Journal of Health Education, 25*, 136-141.

8. Scapp, R. (1993). Feeling the weight of the world (studies) on my shoulders. *The Social Studies, 84*, 67-70.

9. Society for Public Health Education. (1987). SOPHE code of ethics. *Health Education Quarterly, 14*, 79-90.

10. Association for the Advancement of Health Education. (1994). Code of ethics for health educators. *Journal of Health Education, 25*, 196-200.

11. Brookins-Fisher, J., & Rieckmann, T. (1996). The presence of multiculturalism in titles of selected health education journal articles. *The Health Educator, 28*, 3-7.

Chapter 15

BALANCING THE MULTIPLE ROLES OF A HEALTH EDUCATOR

Denise R. Cyzman, M.S., R.D., C.H.E.S.

Author's Comments: *I love my profession! One of the reasons why is because I can always count on my job, as a health education specialist, to involve a wide variety of roles and responsibilities. Although many of the positions I have held call upon expertise in using similar health education skills and competencies, the variety in the positions is such that I have never become bored or complacentæthere is always something new to do. Variety, however, can also be a double-edged sword. Without appropriate direction and focus, variety can lead to work loads that are overwhelming and uncontrollable.*

Being able to effectively live with this double-edged sword over the last 15 years is the reason why I was enthusiastic about writing this chapter. Although practicing many of the strategies outlined in this chapter has become second nature, it can be easy to forget what needs to be done in order to continue working at an efficient and effective level. This is often true when the strategies need to be used the most, that is, when I am the busiest or facing numerous barriers. I have also found that when a balance in professional life is achieved, it is easier to find a balance in my personal and family life. Furthermore, in many of the areas where I need improvement at home, many of the strategies used to strike balance at work can be easily translated to aid in finding balance at home.

When reading this chapter, it is important for you to consider what strategies need to be developed in order for you to maintain balance. Realize that these strategies will change over time as you face new challenges and opportunities. It is through learning how to balance the variety of roles and responsibilities we encounter that we can assure that, as health educators, we play a vital role in the health arena of the future.

INTRODUCTION

Health educators cover the entire health continuum, from helping individuals achieve optimal health, to preventing and controlling disease. The work of health educators is carried out in many settings, involves many responsibilities, and is positioned at various levels within organizations.

With such wide variations in roles and the accompanying responsibilities, it is crucial for current and future health educators to learn how to achieve balance in their jobs. They must be able to perform their duties, use skills and expertise appropriately, maintain efficiency and effectiveness, and overcome barriers that impede their ability to succeed. To do so, while continuing professional growth and development and maintaining a proactive role in the evolving health paradigm, is the real challenge.

Health educators' roles are largely defined by their level and type of position, responsibilities, settings in which they work, and where they work within the organization. It is accurate to say that no two health educator roles are exactly alike, making the number of roles numerous. Determining a health educator's role is similar to identifying the role of a musician. A health educator could be (e.g.) an HIV/AIDS specialist, teacher, or supervisor of a health department. Similarly, a musician could be (e.g.) a pianist, member of a barbershop quartet, or orchestra conductor. A band analogy can be used to describe the four types of roles health educators most often play. In particular, a health educator functions as a (1) solo act, (2) member of a small group or duet, (3) member of a band, or (4) band director.

A *solo act* exists when there is only one health educator in the organization, such as a school health education coordinator at an intermediate school district. This individual must have knowledge and competencies necessary to perform a wide range of health education responsibilities, including: (1) assessing needs; (2) planning, implementing, and evaluating individual and group behavior change programs; (3) coordinating service delivery; (4) serving as a resource person; and (5) communicating needs, concerns, and resources.[1] Because this type of health educator usually operates in isolation, professional networking and collaboration among other staff, key community leaders, and other health and service providers is both necessary and beneficial.

A *duet*, or small group, consists of two or more health educators who either function together in a centralized health education unit or are decentralized in various areas throughout the organization. As with the solo performer, these educators must be well versed in health education theory and practice and demonstrate competence in many areas. They may be more specialized than the generalist solo performer. The more typical scenario, however, involves these educators as generalists, perhaps with a subarea of expertise, who work together to provide well-coordinated services and programs. An outpatient health education specialist and a certified diabetes educator working at a local hospital are examples of two health educators working in this capacity.

A *member of a band* is located in an organization that has many health educators who often work together in a centralized unit. In some cases, they may be spread out and decentralized throughout the organization, and are usually specialized in relation to a specific topic or a narrow set of health education responsibilities. A cancer public education specialist, abstinence coordinator, HIV/AIDS trainer, substance abuse communicable disease specialist, and community planner at a state or local health department is an example of health educators working together as a centralized unit. By having educators with different specialties, the organization can ensure many areas of expertise are available. Coordination and collaboration are key to avoid maximizing organizational effectiveness, which holds true whether the band is in a centralized health education unit or decentralized throughout the organization.

The *band director* is defined as a supervisor, manager, or director of a program or unit. This individual administers, directs, coordinates, manages, evaluates, and supervises health educators and other staff, programs, activities, and budgets. In some cases, these responsibilities go beyond health education and can encompass other professional areas of expertise, such as nursing, epidemiology, and nutrition. Minimal direct service or entry-level responsibilities are seen at this level, although past experience and current knowledge of these responsibilities are needed for effective management. Professional collaborative efforts focus on networking with other supervisors, managers, and directors, regardless of their education, training, or experience. Contrary to the prior three levels, in which positions evolve from general to more specialized, the director reverts to a generalist, with a subspecialty focusing on management or leadership.

The work setting also helps define the roles of the health educator. Health education is delivered in almost every conceivable setting, including schools, health departments, community agencies, worksites, churches, universities, managed-care organizations, hospitals, and private and public physician offices and clinics. The health educator who functions in the entrepreneurial setting or as consultant is also becoming increasingly popular.

Definitions of roles are impacted by work settings largely because the setting dictates that certain responsibilities are carried out. For example, health educators in community settings resolve individual and community health issues by becoming involved in the development of community partnerships, community organization, and individual or group behavior change.[2,3] School health educators engage children and adults at school by involving classroom teaching, teacher training, and changes in the school environment to support health behaviors.[3,4] Worksite and occupational health educators, or health promotion specialists, foster social support, develop worksite norms, and encourage individual behavior change. Their efforts ultimately impact health care costs, morale, productivity, absenteeism, image, and profitability.[3-5] Health education in the health care setting, often referred to as patient education, involves strategies to prevent or detect disease as well as manage acute and chronic illness to maintain or improve health, prevent illness, or slow the progression of disease in patients.[3,4] The variations in roles due to setting orientation hold true regardless of whether the health educator is a solo act, member of a team, or the leader of the band. Regardless of the position, all health educators should be well versed in the major responsibilities and competencies as identified by the National Commission for Health Education Credentialing (NCHEC).[1]

COMMON BARRIERS THAT IMPEDE FULFILLING ROLES AND RESPONSIBILITIES

As in any position, barriers that prevent health educators from fulfilling their roles are numerous. Common barriers that health educators encounter are associated with (1) politics, (2) bureaucracies, (3) lack of resources, (4) interpersonal and interagency conflict, (5) community resistance, (6) personal beliefs, and (7) limitations of research findings. It is important that health educators understand the prevalence and magnitude of these barriers and the strategies for overcoming them.

Politics

Political barriers include (1) official and legislative priorities, (2) changing organizational priorities, and (3) intra-agency politics. These barriers, typically beyond the control of the health educator, can have a tremendous impact on the ability to implement an effective and efficient program or service.

Political and legislative priorities may stray from actual determined needs or professional opinion. For example, the federal, state, or county government may not support use of government funds for needle exchange and other harm reduction programs for HIV/AIDS prevention. While significant research findings and practical application may show that these types of programs are effective in reducing the transmission of HIV among high-risk groups, the political climate or legislative mandate would make it impossible for a government-employed health educator to support implementation of these programs. In cases like this, the health educator is prevented from implementing an effective program. Political priorities that require the educator to "speak the party line," are often demoralizing, but may be overcome as the political climate changes.

In times of rapid change, organizational priorities may change quickly and drastically. For example, a new hospital CEO may determine that the existing senior citizen health screening program should be terminated and a new worksite health promotion program should be initiated. Whether the reason for the shift in priorities is deemed reasonable or unreasonable, it is imperative that the health educator understand the premise for the change, is open to new possibilities, participates proactively in assisting with the change, and exhibits the flexibility necessary to make changes from the existing program to a new one.

Intra-agency politics may create barriers to coordinating or collaborating between similar efforts, and result in a decrease or delay in programs or services delivered. Coordination or collaboration may be impaired when two agency sections have conflicting or varying policies that impact upon program or service implementation. For example, the administration of a large company may ask their health promotion program to provide a health screening that will reach 75% of employees. They will not, however, allow employees to participate in the screening during work time. This conflicts with the health promotion program's plan to implement a comprehensive health screening which takes 30 minutes. Because the screening requires 15 more minutes than the employee's break time, the administration and health promotion program may have difficulty implementing the screening and reaching their targeted goal.

In some cases, intra-agency politics can undermine the ability to provide a program or service in a timely manner or even at all. If, for example, a group of hospital physicians feels that an annual community health screening, sponsored by the hospital health promotion department, would result in their patients not seeking regular medical care, they may apply pressure to hospital administration to stop the event.

Resources

Budget and other programmatic resources greatly influence program impact and outcome measures. Funding amounts are generally not large enough, making it difficult to implement all the programs and services necessary to truly impact the problem. In addition, existing funding levels are often in jeopardy, with real or perceived cuts being common, regardless of the source of funding. As a result, health educators are continually required to justify costs and seek new funding avenues in order to maintain program operation (see Chapter 12, "Grant Writing"). Programmatic resources such as staff, secretarial support, computers, educational materials, and outreach activities may also impact upon the program's success. Without a blend of adequate funding and resources, it is unlikely that the program will reach its full potential in meeting program impact and outcome goals. These funding and resource issues constantly place demands on health educators and reduce time available for other responsibilities (e.g., delivery of health education services).

Bureaucracies

In some large organizations with complex bureaucratic procedures associated with resource allocation, it is difficult to complete tasks. For example, the numerous procedures and rules that may need to be followed to hire new staff may mean that it takes three to six months to fill a vacant position. Bureaucratic procedures associated with purchase procedures, agreements, or contracts may increase the time it takes from ordering supplies or equipment to delivery of these items. Procedures or policies like these make it difficult for a health educator to be efficient and effective in carrying out day-to-day responsibilities. In addition, organizational downsizing or "rightsizing"—having to do more with less resources—is the status quo and can be an obstacle that affects not only one's ability to perform, but also morale and commitment.

Interpersonal and Interagency Conflicts

Because differing interests or priorities are common, interpersonal or interagency conflict may result when (1) individuals or organizations have the same or similar goals but differ on approaches or methods, (2) problem-solving priorities and values differ, and (3) "turf" issues exist. These conflicts are unlikely to go away on their own, and until addressed may impede the health educator's ability to be able to meet responsibilities efficiently and effectively. The following examples, although all specific to interagency conflict, illustrate these three types of interpersonal or interagency conflict.

1. Planning agencies and the Right to Life movement have the same goal—to prevent unwanted pregnancy and decrease abortions—but have different thoughts on how to reach this goal.

2. Two agency programs may need to fight for limited funding because of pending funding cuts. One program focuses on cancer prevention and the other focuses on HIV/AIDS prevention, resulting in pitting the importance of cancer prevention against the importance of HIV/AIDS prevention.

3. Two agencies are unwilling to work together to coordinate a community screening because neither agency wants to share credit for involvement.

Community Resistance

Community resistance may also occur for the same reasons listed in the previous section, with the conflict existing between the community and the agency. The community may be defined in many ways, including as a group (1) living in a specific geographic area, (2) being served by the same government entity, (3) being of the same racial or ethnic background, or (4) sharing common interests or having other common bonds. Two examples of community resistance include a group of parents who do not wish to have a school-based sexuality education program, and a community that wishes their local community center would use a foundation grant to implement an after-school recreation program rather than provide traditional substance abuse prevention education to high-risk teens.

Personal Beliefs

As in intra-agency, interpersonal, and interagency conflicts, health educators may have similar conflicts between themselves and their agencies or programs. Health educators come to the work setting with their own set of values, beliefs, attitudes, and priorities. These reflect personal growth and development and relate to numerous factors, including cultural background, religion, socioeconomic status, educational background, and prior or current relationships. As such, it would be difficult for health educators to completely "turn off" their personal beliefs that may conflict with the agency or program goals, objectives, or priorities. When faced with such conflicts, the health educator must (1) assess the extent to which the agency's focus varies from the personal belief; (2) determine the possibility of changes in either the agency's focus or the belief; (3) identify strategies to cope with the discrepancy; (4) seek resources in assisting with coping, as necessary; and (5) if the conflict is great enough with no possibility of resolution, identify if the need to seek employment in another agency or program is necessary. An example of such conflict could arise with a Catholic health educator, who believes in "right to life," working at a family planning clinic where abortion is offered as a means of terminating unwanted pregnancies. Another example of a potential conflict could exist with a health educator, who was sexually abused as a child, working in a sexual offender rehabilitation program. It is necessary for health educators to anticipate conflicts both prior to accepting and throughout employment in order to address these conflicts and respond accordingly.

Limitations of Research Findings

Health education and health behavior is a relatively new profession. In comparison to other fields, health education research is limited. This may be due in part to health education research being psychosocial and behavioral in nature, which allows for limitations in drawing exact conclusions. For example, because of the existence of numerous external variables that cannot be controlled, it is very difficult to attribute a community-wide reduction in adolescent sexual behavior to a school-based sexuality education program. It becomes difficult to ascertain the long-term impact attributed directly to health education interventions, making program planning and implementation a challenge. In addition to lack of exactness in health education research, findings continue to evolve over time, requiring continual study and clarification. Although the breadth of health education research is growing, health educators continue to experience difficulty in identifying those approaches that do make a difference.

OVERCOMING BARRIERS

Specific barriers are destined to change over time and are unique to individual situations and settings. As a result, no one can develop a cookbook on how to meet every challenge and overcome all barriers. There are, however, increasing materials to assist health educators in meeting the barriers faced on a daily basis. In general, overcoming barriers requires optimism, a willingness to meet challenges head on, an interest in seeing all sides of an issue, and an ability to be creative in identifying solutions. A simplified framework for overcoming barriers includes (1) identifying potential barriers when planning—being proactive; (2) identifying several creative solutions to the barriers; (3) identifying consequences to each of the potential solutions; and (4) picking the best solution and trying it out—multiple times, if needed. Examples of barriers common to health educators and possible solutions for overcoming them are presented in Tables 15-1 and 15-2.

FINDING BALANCE

Because the roles of health educators are broad and varied, it is critical that a balance exists in order to effectively and efficiently function. Balancing the myriad of roles and responsibilities is both a delicate and a difficult process that demands a great deal of patience and skill. How effective and efficient individuals are in balancing the different aspects of their jobs depends on their ability to (1) access and utilize available resources, (2) set goals and objectives, (3) identify priorities, (4) develop plans of action, (5) justify services, and (5) use time management and time allocation skills consistently.

Accessing and Utilizing Available Resources

Having an understanding of available resources can assist the health educator in knowing what can be done and in what time frame. Rather than getting caught in an "I can do it all" trap, health educators need to understand that numerous resources exist. When used appropriately, these re-

Table 15-1. Barriers and Possible Solutions

Barrier	Possible Solutions
Downsizing or reorganization	1. Get better at adapting. 2. Instead of seeing change as an adversary, accommodate it, align with it, and use it. 3. See how your strengths will benefit the new environment.[8]
Lack of administrative support	1. Provide administrators with information that shows how your program or activity supports the mission of the parent organization or agency.[9]
Community resistance	1. Set alliances with key community leaders. 2. Include community members in the planning. 3. Listen to community concerns and address them. 4. Pilot programs which may be controversial. 5. Provide constant feedback on progress to the community. 6. Evaluate and prove success.
Physician resistance	1. Involve physicians in all levels of program planning—from beginning to eventual evaluation.[10] 2. Show how your programs can enhance their ability to practice efficiently and effectively.
Lack of political support	1. Understand and use power, influence, and persuasion to organize the community to effectively present needs to elected or appointed officials. A large number of people speaking with a unified voice to educate officials creates power, and, therefore, is likely to make an impact in the political arena.[11]

sources can improve effectiveness and efficiency by alleviating both time and skill constraints. The following questions are pertinent to resource identification:

- How much staff time and other resources are really available?
- What outside resources are available for help?
- What financial and other constraints exist?

Resources may be found internally or externally. Internal resources may be identified by considering other staff areas of expertise, job descriptions, time constraints, and willingness to undertake new challenges. Other internal resources include office and computer equipment, health references and educational materials, supplies, and materials. Technological resources such as fax machines, high quality photocopiers, computers, printers, and scanners are particularly helpful. If possible, computer capability should include word processing, desktop publishing, data compilation and analysis, e-mail, and use of the Internet. External resources

Table 15-2. Barriers and Possible Solutions

Barrier	*Possible Solutions*
Intra-agency conflict	1. Develop ongoing relationships with key agency decision makers and individuals from partnering sections. 2. Educate all on the value of the program and what is needed to be done to maintain effectiveness and efficiency. 3. Focus on common goals and collaborative ways to achieve those goals. 4. Involve all in the planning of the program.
Funding cuts on programs	1. Create a unified front on the importance of both programs, regardless of whether they are within the same agency focus. 2. Educate decision-makers on their value and refuse to pit programs against each other. 3. Remain consistent on information presented by both programs and advocate for full funding for both. 4. Emphasize how both programs impact the community.
Delay in hiring staff due to bureaucratic procedures	1. Anticipate the lag time needed to fill positions. 2. Seek short-term solutions with temporary or contractual employees. 3. Adjust work load among remaining staff. 4. Keep informed of the status of the position as it goes through the agency.
Inadequate equipment	1. Identify other equipment within the agency that may be borrowed or shared resources. 2. Identify outside resources that may have equipment available for use or loan. 3. Inform key decision-makers of the need for equipment, especially as it relates to effectiveness and efficiency. 4. Seek additional funding or donations.

may be similar to those listed above, but may be offered by an outside agency as part of a collaborative partnership or given as an in-kind donation. Other external resources may be found by seeking specialty services not available through the agency such as graphic design, public relations, medical care, or computer programming. Funding resources may be obtained, indirectly, through donation of in-kind staff, services, or supplies; mini-grants or donations from local groups or foundations; or defined partnerships with identified sharing of resources.

Identification of resources, whether internal or external, occurs through a continual process. One of the first steps is to be aware of the agency and its programs and staff. By doing so, it will become more apparent where natural intra-agency cooperative efforts or sharing of resources could occur. Secondly, knowing the community and its resources is essential. Networking with similar agency staff, meeting with key community leaders, and discussions with members from the target population help to uncover where resources are and where they are lacking. Finally, printed community directories, such as community service directories and the telephone book may be helpful in giving the health educator a start toward resource identification.

Setting Goals

To work effectively and efficiently, the health educator must have direction for what should and can be done. Setting goals and accompanying objectives provides this by defining the purpose, or direction, of the program and recognizing what can be accomplished. To help the health educator have a clear direction, goals and objectives should be specific, measurable, and realistic. General goals and objectives are not useful to the health educator as they do not spotlight the path, nor allow assessment of progress toward being effective and efficient in meeting the program purpose. Similarly, overly optimistic goals and objectives are self-defeating and set up for failure.

Without goals and objectives, decisions and actions may be driven externally or grow out of control, thus keeping the health educator off balance and moving in a direction away from their purpose. For example, the health educator may be implementing activities to reduce the prevalence of diabetes among Hispanics. Halfway through the year, the administration may ask the educator to plan and implement a violence prevention media campaign targeting African-Americans. While both efforts may be worthwhile and necessary, having previously defined goals and objectives related to diabetes allows the health educator to question the rationale for the request and assess the impact this change would have on reaching the previously set goals and objectives. This type of discussion helps others to realize the impact that the deviation could have on the ability to achieve previously set targets. As a result, a decision to stay with activities to reach previously set goals and objectives is often made. On rarer occasions, the change is determined necessary, especially when previously set goals and objectives may no longer be feasible or appropriate.[6] Regardless of the result of the discussion, evaluating proposed changes will force decisions to be driven with careful thought and consideration and enable the health educator to continue to proceed in a clearly defined fashion.

Identifying Priorities

Priorities focus on what is truly important. Identifying priorities helps to define a workable schedule for accomplishing tasks and are based upon program goals.[7] Knowing priorities and sticking to them, however, are not one in the same. Because of numerous and sometimes conflicting responsibilities, it is easy to be pulled in different directions, have priorities moved to the back burner, or to have priorities that conflict. If this happens, it is likely that the balance necessary for effectiveness and efficiency will not occur. Thus, to stay focused, the following questions should be considered:

- How does this project or request fit in with personal and professional priorities?

- Is it appropriate to assume responsibility for this task?

- What impact will diverting time have on accomplishing other tasks or meeting other deadlines?

- Can this problem be solved by others, and if so, by whom?

Identification of and remaining focused on priorities helps the health educator work in a manner that is most effective and efficient in achieving goals and objectives by avoiding detours into areas that are not crucial.

Developing Plans of Action

Developing a plan of action is the process of establishing workable time frames to ensure that goals and objectives are achieved. This plan, based upon previously set goals, objectives and priorities, helps to maintain balance by identifying pathways to effectively and efficiently accomplish tasks. The tasks in the plan illuminate the pathways by specifying what needs to be done to meet goals and objectives. The time frames set realistic deadlines and give the health educator a clearly defined schedule from which to work.

Plans can be simple in format or very complex, with the level of detail dependent on the needs of the health educator and the organization.

When determining the necessary level of detail, the plan needs to maintain its ability to be a management tool, rather than a tool that manages the individual. A poorly written or, lack of, a plan of action may detract from engaging in the work necessary to accomplish tasks and, reach goals and objectives.

Many templates for plans of action have been developed. The following are examples of three different formats, ranging from simple to more complex. All three examples relate to the same goal and corresponding objective.

Example Action Plans

Goal:	By the year 2000, reduce the incidence of diabetes among Michigan Hispanics from 12,000 to 10,000.
Objective:	By September 30, 1997, identify three culturally sensitive and appropriate strategies for providing diabetes prevention to Hispanics with diabetes.

Example 1

Tasks:	1.	Identify existing prevention materials and other resources that have been developed and used for Hispanics.
	2.	Prepare a draft resource list of existing materials and resources.

Example 2

Task	Responsible Party	Target Date	Status
Identify existing prevention materials and other resources that have been developed and used for Hispanics.	Courtney Smith	9/1/97	Finished
Prepare a draft resource list of existing materials and resources.	Courtney Smith; Ryan Jones	9/15/97	Pending

Example 3

Task	Key Players	Other Resources	Time Allotment	Target Date
Identify existing prevention materials and other resources that have been developed and used for Hispanics.	Courtney Smith	CDC, Other State Diabetes Programs, Diabetes Outreach Networks	80 hours	9/1/97
Prepare a draft resource list of existing materials and resources.	Courtney Smith; Ryan Jones	Sample Materials, Word Processor, Supervisor Review	20 hours	9/9/97

Justifying Services

Evaluation is critical in helping educators keep a balance, as results show the degree to which efforts are effective and efficient. Without evaluation, health educators would be unlikely to know program outcomes or unable to justify their work. The purpose of evaluation is to assess effectiveness and efficiency by answering three questions:[4]

- Are we doing the best we can with the resources that we have?

- Is the program/intervention having any effect?

- So what?

The first question deals with efficiency, and focuses on process evaluation. It is designed to assess whether resources, including the health educator's time, are being efficiently and effectively used. The second question relates to program effectiveness and focuses on impact evaluation. The third question addresses outcome evaluation and identifies whether changes have made a difference in health status (e.g., morbidity, mortality, and disability). In essence, program evaluation can help health educators in balancing their multiple roles and responsibilities by assisting in recognizing and prioritizing skills and resources to be used.

Because evaluation is an integral part of program development and implementation, analyses and documentation of results are crucial. Only through documentation will health educators show that working efficiently and effectively produces impact and outcome changes, regardless of availability of resources. Documenting evaluation results are important for three reasons: (1) To verify that the program *did* make a difference, (2) to identify revisions (including resource and personnel allocations) that are necessary, and (3) to show others that the program *can* make a difference. Personal evaluation efforts may also focus on the ability and competencies of the health educator to adequately meet their responsibilities. These efforts are also important to see whether or not the match between the health educator, program, and target audience is working. Often this type of evaluation includes personal skill or knowledge assessments, supervisory observation or periodic staff evaluation, and review of program process and outcome evaluation results by the individual educator.

Once evaluation efforts show the effectiveness and efficiency of the health educator and / or the service, it is necessary to share these with key decision-makers. Documenting and sharing results, as an ongoing method to justify the service is necessary, *even if not asked to do so*. Results should be shared with administrators, funders, program participants, the community, legislators, and local, state and federal officials. These results should (1) be in reports prepared on a regular basis (e.g., at least annually); (2) include process, impact, and outcome evaluation measures; and (3) be reader friendly and appropriate for the target audience. While it is tempting to share with others all that is known about or has been collected on a program, information is only useful to the reader if it answers the question, "What will show *me* that you are successful?"

Managing and Allocating Time

One of the major constraints to balancing the many roles and responsibilities associated with health education is having enough time to effectively accomplish tasks and assignments. Even with the best plans, balancing time will, at some point, be a problem. Time management and allocation skills can assist health educators in becoming more efficient and effective in juggling their numerous commitments.

Time management uses a group of guidelines to structure time that is spent on various activities in order to improve efficiency. In contrast, time allocation involves setting priorities to determine which tasks need to be completed and in what order.[7] Tips and techniques used in time management and allocation are numerous, with many books, planners, tapes, conferences, and seminars available as guides. Some of the more helpful techniques are presented in Table 15-3.

Along with incorporating time management and allocation practices, it is important to learn how to say no. Although many people find this difficult, it is often the appropriate response and will usually be accepted by others. Similar to steps used for prioritization, it is important to (1) think about whether a request fits within personal and professional goals and priorities, (2) determine who is the best person for the job, (3) suggest other possible solutions or alternatives, (4) ask if it is possible to help on a limited basis, (5) define what one can and cannot do, and (6) understand that

Table 15-3. Time Management Techniques

- Using goals and objectives to set priorities and then staying focused on the priorities.

- Breaking larger tasks into smaller, more manageable tasks.

- Developing a plan and setting, or negotiating, realistic deadlines.

- Using meetings wisely—being action oriented with specific results expected.

- Turning idle time into productive time—using time waiting for phone calls or traveling to read mail, scan articles or other paperwork, return low priority phone calls, write short memos or correspondence, and file.

- Avoiding reinventing the wheel—seeing what has already been done to determine how it can be used or adapted.

- Organizing work space by creating a system with everything at easy access.

- Delegating and working with others, especially focusing on each other's strengths and dividing tasks accordingly.

- Learning to be proactive by focusing on what is important rather than urgent.

saying no does not cause bad feelings nor does saying yes win a popularity contest or ensure career advancement.

Key to time management and allocation processes is taking the time needed to organize. Without taking time to organize, more time is spent without a focus, engaging in activities that have no impact on the final outcome, and searching for needed items or materials.

Finally, even with numerous time management and allocation techniques available, being flexible is important. Sometimes, no matter how carefully time is planned, an event or "opportunity" happens that supersedes time management efforts and forces deviation from the path. Learning to cope with these fluctuations while still remaining flexible is essential for completing tasks and avoiding burnout.

PREPARING FOR THE FUTURE THROUGH CONTINUED EDUCATION

Because health education is continually expanding, education and learning does not stop with graduation and job orientation. As with other fields and professions, continuing education is a natural extension to formal education. In determining which type of continuing education is appropriate, a number of options should be explored. The typical and most common types of continuing education activities include conferences, trainings, teleconferences, and university courses. Even though these activities are widely available, they may not be as easily accessible. For instance, health educators in rural settings may be unable to take advantage of advanced training because of limited financial resources or geographic constraints.

The latest information on programmatic results and theory application is often released through journals (e.g., *Journal of School Health, Health Education & Behavior, Journal of Health Education, American Journal of Public Health*), text books, and other written resources. Many of these publications offer opportunities for continuing education creditæincluding Certified Health Education Specialist (CHES) creditæwhich may alleviate problems associated with accessibility. In addition, advancements in computer technology provide unlimited opportunities to expand the scope of knowledge. The Internet, electronic mail, distance learning, and innovative software programs provide immediate information about the latest scientific findings, program updates, and advice from colleagues. Health educators can also learn from each other. Networking and sharing is, and will continue to be, one of the most effective and efficient ways to learn how to better programs, implement new services, and utilize previously unknown resources.

The National Commission for Health Education Credentialing has established a national certification process (i.e., CHES) designed to certify health education specialists, promote professional development, and strengthen professional preparation. This entry-level certification benefits health educators, employers, and consumers by (1) confirming the educator's minimum knowledge and skill level, (2) helping employers identify qualified applicants, (3) helping consumers recognize services provided by a qualified educator, (4) improving professional practice, and (5) defining the health education scope of practice. The certification requires continuing education credits, which further enhances the ability of the health educator to continue with lifelong learning.

Health educators prepared at the bachelor's level should consider pursuing an advanced degree. In this fast-changing world, postgraduate degrees are becoming necessary for employment, particularly for management and other administrative positions. Choice of an advanced degree is an individual decision, based on interest and impact upon a designated career path. Depending on career path, it may be advantageous to complement the bachelor's degree in health education with a degree in a related field to widen the scope of expertise. An example would be a bachelor's degree in health education, with a master's degree in public health, nursing, health communications, epidemiology, or business. Appropriate fields of study for advanced degrees in fields related to health education are listed in Table 15-4.

Finally, given the current climate of organizational downsizing, agency reorganization, and geographic mobility, changes in employment

Table 15-4. Related Graduate Programs of Study

- Health Education
- Public Health
- Health Communications
- Social Marketing
- Program Evaluation
- Epidemiology
- Nutrition
- Exercise Physiology
- Behavioral Science
- Educational Psychology
- Social Work
- Nursing
- Management
- Marketing
- Public Administration
- Health Care Administration

is increasingly necessary. As such, having a broad base of education, experience, and expertise is recommended for career advancement or mobility. Having professional training or experience in various health-related areas, settings, and positions will provide the health educator with a varied level of expertise. This will only enhance opportunities for job mobility by qualifying for more positions should changes be necessary or desired. Persons limiting their scope of expertise, however, will find it more difficult to find new positions as their choices for available positions may be limited.

WHERE DO WE GO FROM HERE?

As stated by Karen Glanz in *Health Behavior and Health Education,* "Perhaps never before have those concerned with health education been faced with more challenges and opportunities than they are today."[3] The body of knowledge related to health education, largely drawn from scientific and evaluative research, has grown at an exponential rate. Although difficult to draw *exact* conclusions as to the effectiveness of health education practices, many studies have found extremely promising results. Health education programming is, therefore, increasingly seen as a viable means of optimizing health and preventing disease. In addition, the profession is increasingly seen as legitimate and distinct, which is fortified with a national health education certification system. What is needed to maintain the health educator role as an integral component in improving the health of communities rests on the following two questions: (1) How will health educators fit into the evolving world of medical and managed care, worksite, and public health as these change over time? and (2) what should be done to ensure the involvement of health educators remains integral?

Christopher Atchinson summarized some of the major changes in the health of our nation when he suggested: "To deal with chronic disease, we must have a new vision of the vectors; not mosquitoes or rats (the 1800s paradigm) rather behavior—the choices we make; the actions we take."[12] He defined the modern vectors as behaviors—individual and community—that "carry" chronic disease. Rather than accept chronic disease as inevitable, there must be awareness that individuals and communities can make changes, that movement must occur from physical to behavioral conditions, and health educators must motivate and facilitate positive health behaviors.[12] At the same time, the role of public health is in a period of flux. Core public health functions have been defined as assessment, policy development, and assurance (see Chapter 1, "Community Health Assessment and Improvement"). These core public health functions require an understanding of health surveillance; epidemiology; social and behavioral science; data collection and its use in program planning, implementation, and development; and policy development.[13]

Taking all this into consideration, it is now time for health educators to take a good look at their roles and, if necessary, refine them to ensure that they are integrated into the evolving health care and public health paradigm. As stated previously, qualified health educators are educated and trained to (1) assess needs; (2) plan, implement, and evaluate individual and group behavior change programs; (3) coordinate service delivery; (4) serve as resource persons; and (5) communicate needs, concerns, and resources.[1] Following the rules identified in Osborne's *Reinventing Government*, health educators can assist in this process by (1) making efforts proactive—steering rather than rowing; (2) empowering the community to be active, rather than passive, and to help define what is needed and how it should be implemented; (3) developing programs and services that meet organizational missions; (4) assuring that results are collected and analyzed—focusing on outcomes rather than inputs; and (5) keeping the focus on prevention rather than cure.[14]

The roles of the health educator fit perfectly with the evolving health care system. The knowledge, competencies, and job responsibilities are all defined to help communities, individuals, and the nation maximize their health through behavioral and environmental changes that promote optimal health and prevent disease. Health educators are charged, therefore, with refining their roles and organizing as a profession to market them. To do so, they must build alliances in the public and private sector so that strategies are rich and deep and likelihood of success is high. Health educators must be at the forefront of helping others see how they can and must play integral roles in the ever-changing health paradigm.

References

1.   National Task Force on the Preparation and Practice of Health Educators. (1990). *A framework for the development of competency-based curricula for entry-level health educators.* New York: National Commission for Health Education Credentialing, Inc.

2.   Joint Committee on Health Education Terminology. (1991). Report of the 1990 Joint Committee on Health Education Terminology. *Journal of Health Education, 22,* 173-184.

3.   Glanz, K., Lewis, F. M., & Rimer, B. (Eds). *Health behavior and health education: Theory, research, and practice.* San Francisco: Jossey-Bass.

4.   Deeds, S. G. (1992). *The health education specialist.* Los Alamitos, CA: Loose Canon Publications.

5.   O'Donnell, M. P., & Harris, J. S. (Eds.). (1994). *Health promotion in the workplace* (2nd ed.). Albany, NY: Delmar Publishers.

6.   Pell, A. R. (1995). *The complete idiot's guide to managing people.* New York: Alpha Books.

7.   Brewer, K. C. (1991). *Getting things done.* Shawnee Mission, KS: National Press Publications.

8.   Pritchett, P., & Pound, R. (1995). *The stress of organizational change.* Dallas: Pritchett & Associates.

9.   Dhillon, H. S, & Tolsma D. (1988). *Meeting global health challenges: A position paper on health education.* Atlanta: Centers for Disease Control and Prevention.

10.   Krenaghan, S. G, & Giloth, B. E. (1983). *Working with physicians in health promotion.* Chicago: American Hospital Publishing Company.

11.   Breckon, D. (1990). Using politics to affect health education policy at the local level. *Community organization: Traditional principles and modern application.* Johnson City, TN: Latchpins Press.

12.   Atchinson, C. (1993). How can ASTHO and public health nutritionists continue the process. *Proceedings: Celebrating the past, shaping the future.* Minneapolis: University of Minnesota.

13.   Institute of Medicine. (1988). *The future of public health.* Washington, DC: National Academy Press.

14.   Osborne, D., & Gaebler, T. (1993). *Reinventing government: How the entrepreneurial spirit is transforming the public sector.* New York: Penguin Books.

Chapter 16

THE FUTURE OF LOCAL PUBLIC HEALTH EDUCATION

Richard M. Tooker, M.D., M.P.H.

Author's Comments: *As I was writing this chapter, it occurred to me that I have actually achieved a measure of wisdom through years of practical experience in public health. As a physician, one would expect me to be a skilled educator. Any physician should be. This, however, is not often the case. There is a tremendous need for well-educated health educators to join in partnership with health care providers. It is also time for our health care to embrace the formal skills of the health educator. The chapters contained in this book should be standard reading for all health-related professionals, including health educators, doctors, nurse practitioners, physician's assistants, nurses, and other traditional health care providers. We all need to speak the language and understand the application of preventive health education. It works at any level of health promotion and health care intervention.*

INTRODUCTION

The role and mission of public health has always been to prevent disease, protect the public's health, and provide preventive and personal health services. As the new century progresses, local public health will undergo transformations that will parallel health care reform. As summarized by Vernice Davis Anthony, then Vice-President of Community and Urban Affairs for St. John Health System:

> *Health and quality of life for citizens will occur only with a continued complementary interaction between the medical care and public health care systems. Essential parts of the new system are population-based services and a state and local governmental presence in assessing the health needs of the population, preventing disease and disability, promoting and protecting the public's health, and providing access to needed services.*

Local public health educators in communities across the United States will be part of an evolutionary process that will place them firmly at the center of a new health care delivery system. New roles and responsibilities may well place the local health educator in a pivotal position not unlike the traditional health care practitioner. The importance of promoting health, preventing disease, protecting populations from harm, and maximizing an individual's potential is becoming the ultimate mission of a reformed health care system. The United States, by pure necessity, is transforming from primarily a sick-care system to a true health maintenance system.

It has been well established in the closing decades of the 20th century that governments, institutions, or business and industry alone cannot solve problems. Only communities, by and through the collaborative involvement of citizens, will exact long-term and meaningful change. This alone establishes the local public health educator in a most exciting and fulfilling role for the future.

The future of local public health has been mapped out in key documents such as *The Future of Public Health, Healthy People 2000,* and *Healthy Communities 2000.*[1-3] These documents define a new and seamless integration of public health and traditional medical care to achieve an optimal state of health for all community residents. Local public health is no longer the exclusive domain of the federal, state, and local health departments. Rather, public health is truly becoming community-owned. Local public health will continue to have government sponsorship to provide for population-based health practices, to provide regulatory authority where needed, and to sponsor direct services the community deems appropriate.

As discussed in Chapter 1, the health educator of the future will find local public health invested in a continuous process of assessment, policy development, assurance, and evaluation.[1] These population-based practices rely upon scientific and epidemiologic investigation to profile the community's health status. The details of these assessments then drive the development of policy to address identified problems. Local public health, in partnership with an array of community health care providers, may then most effectively provide services that will produce healthy communities.

The future vision and mission of local public health may be summarized as follows: Public health serves as the central organization for the application of the values, practices, and principles of health promotion, disease prevention, personal protection, and social justice. These activities will serve to ensure the vitality, longevity, and well-being for all members of the community.

HEALTH EDUCATION: THE FOUNDATION FOR POPULATION-BASED HEALTH CARE

The future mission of local public health presents the health educator with fertile ground to participate in the entire range of the practitioner's responsibilities and competencies as required for certification.[4] Improving the overall health of the public will involve increasing degrees of collaboration with community health providers. The majority of skills and competencies outlined in this book will be utilized by the local health educator in support of the core functions of public health.

The health educator is the most skilled health professional for effective interagency communication, translation of complex health and medical information for the public, and the facilitation of successful applications of important information. Local public health often relies on the health educator to develop communications for the entire population or selected vulnerable, high-risk populations. Public health will, however, continue to need the expertise of the health educator in one-on-one communications. A specific look at the core functions of local public health will help illustrate the application of the health educator's skills.

Assessment

As detailed in Chapter 1, a comprehensive assessment of a community's health should include detailed personal health status indicators. Environmental, social, economic, cultural, and educational characteristics must also be profiled. Advances in technology will provide unlimited information and greater ability to interpret this information. Health educators are vital to this process. For example, an epidemiologist often needs a health educator's participation in the surveillance process and always needs the health educator's skills to package and present data in a useful manner.

Policy Development

Local public health is evolving into the community's central, neutral ground for the maintenance and advancement of planned health programming. Agreed upon health standards are becoming the vision and values of community members more so than ever before. This is reflected in local health policy coordinated by public health departments. Utilizing an understandable community health assessment, the health educator may become a key team member in crafting health policy for community well-being. Coalition building, conducting focus groups, public relations, marketing, mass media and legislative advocacy are tools covered in previous chapters. These tools enable the health educator to contribute to the success of planned interventions for health improvement.

Assurance

For many years local public health has been responsible for population-based health care as well as the added responsibility for direct personal care. In many urban and rural areas, local public health is the only provider of clinical preventive services and primary health care for people lacking access to care. The future health educator will find the assurance of overall community health is a dynamic, ongoing process, owned by every segment of the local community. The future will see less state and federal involvement resulting in the local health department taking a leadership role in the tasks of assurance. Other team members will represent hospitals, health practitioners, schools, nonprofit health agencies, business and industry, courts and law enforcement, churches, and community mental health providers, to name a few. The local health educator will find many important roles in the support of local public health's clinical preventive services (e.g., family planning, health promotion, communicable disease control). The most promising roles for future health educators, however, will be within the rich array of collaboratives, initiatives, and partnerships forming for maximum community health potential. The health educator will be instrumental in the community empowerment process through interpretation, transmission and delivery of health information.

TREND ANALYSIS AND THE FUTURE FOCUS OF LOCAL PUBLIC HEALTH EDUCATION

In looking carefully at the direction of change in communities, trends emerge that help define the future of local public health responsibilities. Universal access to comprehensive health care; the aging of the U.S. population; increasing racial, ethnic and cultural diversity; and the ever-expanding impact of a community upon the land, point to present and future public health challenges. The continued availability of safe food, air, water, and land for our communities will require new partnerships for protection. Environmental safety is increasingly challenged as communities expand across the land. The future will also be about gradual changes in vulnerable populations and how communities assign management of their health needs. Violence and unintentional injuries will continue to be major public health problems. Greater attention will be given to establishing a more peaceful and safe society. Specific examples may help frame future job activities for the health educator and how this profession will fit into the bigger picture.

First, the health educator will have a role in personal preventive health care services. The drive to control health care costs and eventually have affordable health care for all is pushing traditional medical care into the public health prevention frontier. Managed health care plans will need to prevent expensive chronic diseases and disabilities in their enrolled populations as chronic conditions presently affect 90 million Americans at a cost of 659 billion dollars per year.[5]

Health education has had a long history of excellence in controlling and preventing the above diseases in the areas of worksite and community wellness, nutrition, fitness, preventive health screening, and risk reduction counseling. The future health educator in these areas will find their home more in the health maintenance organization than in the health department or hospital. The empowerment of individuals to take responsibility for their health and well-being is essential to the success of our health care system, and will require the blending of quality health education and managed medical care.

Second, there will be an increased need for health promotion programming for older populations as the "baby-boomer" generation ages. The notion of secondary and tertiary prevention suggests a future course for health education. Communities throughout America will need to plan actively for the progressive demographic shift to an older population. It is well recognized that the current traditional health care system is unaffordable. In the very near future, support for traditional Medicare and Medicaid for older Americans will no longer be available. Managed-care plans will be highly motivated to minimize sick-care costs for older adults. The skills of the health educator at the local public health level and at the clinical level will be put to new challenges. How does one achieve a measure of optimum physical, mental, and social function given the natural progression of age? How may one be educated to remain self-sufficient or minimally assisted despite chronic disease? How will health providers and communities evolve to meet the health promotion and disability-minimizing needs of older populations?

Third, health education will have continued involvement in community-based risk assessment and improvement as our nation's demographics change. The local health department will develop an increasing focus on risk for adverse health consequences that may be present at a more encompassing, global level. If, for example, traditional health care providers concentrate on education to increase seat belt use or reduce drinking and driving, then local public health is given the latitude to address such universal risks as poor road design and improved transportation safety. Consensus-building, coalitions, legislative advocacy, and advanced technology in teaching become the hallmark skills of the community health educator in addressing risks for adverse health consequences.

Ultimately, the extension of optimal health to all members of the community will require the interpretation and management of health risk among special community groups. The attainment of health and well-being for underserved individuals will need to be corrected through a community consensus of desire to change the status quo. The reduction of social injustice, classism, greed, and apathy may be aptly called, "pre-primary care." To successfully correct these root causes of disease will reduce the threat to the vitality and survival of the entire community. The local health educator may in the future, be part health expert, part social scientist and part opinion leader in order to make successful pre-primary care a reality.

Last, health education will be necessary in relaying the importance of environmental issues as global changes occur to the detriment of human life. The natural and man-made environments are inherently dangerous. From natural disasters such as floods and earthquakes, to the prevalence of weapons and toxic chemicals, environmental harm causes almost 20% of all deaths. Neither the public nor health care providers typically rate environmental risks as a high priority for health risk reduction. Except at times of episodic harm, will individuals consider the appreciable risk of the physical environment. At other times, the public holds an extremely fearful perception of environmental harm. This may occur even when medical science fails to document even minimal risk. For example, the placement of a sanitary landfill in a community is often an exercise in civic futility because of fearful perceptions alone. Accurate and effective communication of known environmental risk, then, will become a prime task of future local public health educators. Entire communities need enhanced knowledge of potential and actual environmental risk, interpretation of these risks, and understanding of risk abatement strategies. These needs are ideal for the health education practices outlined in this book. The future health educator, working with sophisticated geographic mapping information systems, will be able to actively monitor developing environmental risk and help devise proactive population protection.

Analysis of trends allows a reasonably accurate view of the future for health education. The local health educator in the future will be a highly valuable member in the process of planned, comprehensive community health.

TOWARD COMPREHENSIVE COMMUNITY HEALTH EDUCATION: PUTTING IT ALL TOGETHER

Local public health departments will continue to engage in activities uniquely appropriate for government. A community public health department is acceptable, neutral ground among health care providers, community health agencies, and employers. Local public health is best suited to collect, maintain, and interpret the community health data base. Through their assurance mission, local health departments are ideal leaders in community health improvement efforts.

The National Association of County Health Officials and Centers for Disease Control and Prevention jointly developed *Blueprint for a Healthy Community: A Guide for Local Health Departments*, which lists as one of the

10 essential responsibilities, "mobilizing the community for action."[6] This powerful policy development role has spawned "Healthy Community" initiatives across the country. These new collaboratives in the future may evolve into as yet unknown public or private ventures. Some experts predict that "public health agencies that want to thrive will inevitably transact more of their business through legally constituted partnerships with other public and private entities, as well as through publicly accountable nonprofit corporations (e.g., public benefit corporations)."[7] Health department direct service programs (assurance activities) such as maternal and child health, immunization clinics, and dental public health programs may, in many communities, function very well in managed-care organizations. Communities with fewer provider resources may seek to consolidate local public health into a blended community health provider network.

These visionary statements are the result of health care providers moving beyond isolated programs run from disjointed organizations. Indeed, the future local public health educator may be employed by the health department, but may work in a variety of community health organizations. Progression toward a truly seamless health delivery system, implies a seamless continuum of health education applications. With advanced communication technology in hand, the local public health educator will undoubtedly be linked with health education partners in universities, managed-care organizations, hospitals, clinics, nonprofit agencies, business, and allied government units.

This comprehensive approach to community health is ideally suited to solve multifactorial, refractory health problems such as unintentional injury, domestic and neighborhood violence, substance abuse, and teen pregnancy. The concept of "shared care" is evolving among community health providers and is perhaps most evident in partnerships between public health and the evolving medical care delivery system. Health educators will find the goals of prevention and primary care coming together. Outreach programs, clinical-based practice, and lifelong health education, present an exciting future for the community health educator. From personal health counselor to grant writer to coordinator of community health promotion programs, the future health educator should find everything but boredom. Balancing multiple roles and responsibilities may be one of the greatest skills future health educators can possess.

CONCLUSION

Ultimately, public health is about maximizing potential life span and the compression of morbidity to the farthest possible point on the life line. Communities have a need to enhance the health and well-being of their members. Individuals and families have a need to achieve self-sufficiency and responsibility for healthy behavior. Health education is the language of empowerment and health educators are the translators of health knowledge. The future will bring unlimited health information to almost every individual. The health educator, however, must be the manager of this information for optimum benefit.

Ongoing research is needed to enhance the effectiveness of health education messages. A marriage of research and advanced information technologies may well establish health education as the ultimate vaccine for the multitude of health risks in the 21st century.

References

1. Institute of Medicine. (1988). *The future of public health*. Washington, DC: National Academy Press.

2. Department of Health and Human Services. (1991). *Healthy people 2000: National health promotion and disease prevention objectives*. Washington, DC: U.S. Government Printing Office.

3. The American Public Health Association. (1991). *Healthy communities 2000: Model standards*. Washington, DC: Author.

4. AAHA/SOPHE Joint Committee for the Development of Graduate Level Preparation Standards. (1996). *New responsibilities and competencies*. Washington, DC: Society for Public Health Education.

5. Hoffman, C., Rice D., & Hai-Yen S. (1996). Persons with chronic conditions: Their prevalence and costs, *Journal of the American Medical Association, 276*, 1473-79.

6. National Association of County Health Officials, & Centers for Disease Control and Prevention. (1994). *Blueprint for a healthy community: A guide for local health departments*. Washington, DC: United States Public Health Service.

7. Baker E. L., Melton R. J., Strange P. V., et al. (1994). Health reform and the health of the public. *Journal of the American Medical Association, 272*, 1276-82.